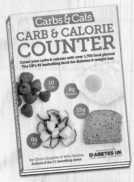

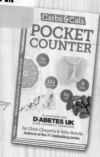
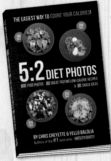
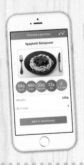
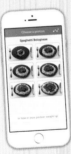

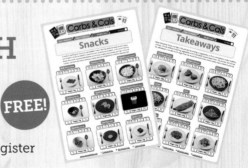

Carbs & Cals VERY LOW CALORIE RECIPES & MEAL PLANS

Lose weight, improve blood sugar levels and reverse type 2 diabetes

1ST EDITION
First published in Great Britain in 2017
by Chello Publishing Limited
Registered Company Number 7237986
www.chellopublishing.co.uk | info@chellopublishing.co.uk
Copyright © Chello Publishing Limited 2017

With special thanks to: Fran Turner, George Malache, Gian Mizzi, Justine Rose, Maxine Gregory, Mike Rogers, Simon Callaghan, Tom Maund, Victoria Francis & Yoshi Balolia.

ISBN: 978-1-908261-20-5 Printed in Malta 0218

Authors	Chris Cheyette BSc (Hons) MSc RD Yello Balolia BA (Hons)
Recipes by	Chris Cheyette BSc (Hons) MSc RD Victoria Francis BSc (Hons) RD
Photography	Simon Callaghan & Francesca Turner
Design Concept	George F Malache
Graphic Design	Maxine Gregory BA (Hons)
Additional Layout	Yello Balolia BA (Hons)
Introduction Text	Victoria Francis BSc (Hons) RD
Assistant Dietitian	Monika Jakiel-Rusin BSc (Hons) MSc RD

For more information, please visit:
www.carbsandcals.com

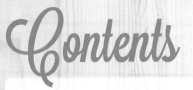

Contents

Introduction

Thank you for choosing **Carbs & Cals VERY LOW CALORIE RECIPES & MEAL PLANS**. This book is a support guide for anyone following a very low-calorie diet approach, such as the Newcastle Low-Calorie Diet Programme or Dr Michael Mosley's 8-Week Blood Sugar Diet. It shows you visually how to create a range of different meal plans for 30 days and beyond.

Have you been told your blood sugar levels are too high (a term coined "pre-diabetes")? Or have you been diagnosed with type 2 diabetes and are keen to halt it in its tracks?

If you are motivated by the idea that changing your eating habits could improve your high blood sugar levels and reverse your diabetes, but the notion of only eating around 800 calories a day feels impossible, then this is the book for you! Specifically designed to help keep you feeling full, our 30 fantastic meal plans (each with around 800 calories per day) will help you plan your low-calorie days, whilst also providing a wide range of nutrients. The book has been developed to give you simple guidance on which foods to include on your shopping list, as well as evidence-based nutrition facts to help you stick to your eating plan.

Fast forward 8 weeks and you've reached your goal... Now what? This book also offers guidance and inspiration on what to choose after 8 weeks to ensure your weight loss journey continues in the longer-term.

What is a very low-calorie diet?

Very low-calorie diets are those that provide up to 800 calories a day, and should be followed for a maximum of 12 weeks. They are not a new idea and have been used for many years. A diet approach using this concept that has made headlines is Dr Michael Mosley's 8-Week Blood Sugar Diet. This is based on evidence from scientific trials carried out at Newcastle University, where research funded by Diabetes UK showed that following a very low-calorie diet for 8 weeks caused significant weight loss, a reduction in the amount of fat in the liver and pancreas, and a restoration of insulin production. This led to reversal of high blood sugar levels in people recently diagnosed with type 2 diabetes.

Participants in the trial (under close medical supervision) followed a strict, low-calorie diet of around 700 calories per day, which consisted of liquid formulated drinks and non-starchy vegetables. Three months after completion of the trial, despite weight gain in some, most participants had normal blood sugar levels.

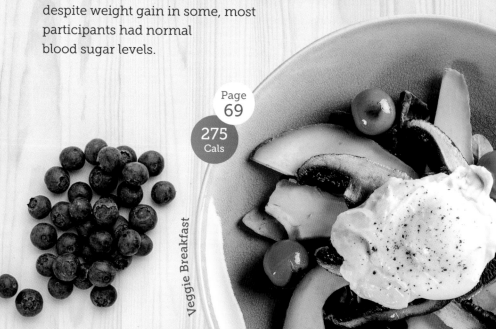

Page
69

275
Cals

Veggie Breakfast

The initial research trial in Newcastle only included a small number of individuals but the findings made national and international headlines, as it was shown that type 2 diabetes could be reversed by diet. One of the key findings was that rapid weight loss depleted fat stores in the liver and pancreas. Large amounts of fat stored in the liver and pancreas (which is one of the main factors that leads to type 2 diabetes) can happen if you are eating and drinking more calories than your body requires. The researchers at Newcastle were clear to point out that the weight loss needs to be sustained in the long term and that this is not just a quick fix. Therefore, what people go on to eat *after* the very low-calorie weight loss plan is equally important.

In 2013, scientists at the Universities of Glasgow and Newcastle were awarded Diabetes UK's largest ever research grant. The purpose of the grant was to study the long-term health effects of following a very low-calorie diet compared to the current care of people with type 2 diabetes, over a five year period. The study is still ongoing but has promising early results. Due to this research, there is growing interest in the use of very low-calorie diets to achieve rapid weight loss and reversal of high blood sugar levels in people with type 2 diabetes, as well as those who may be at risk of developing diabetes.

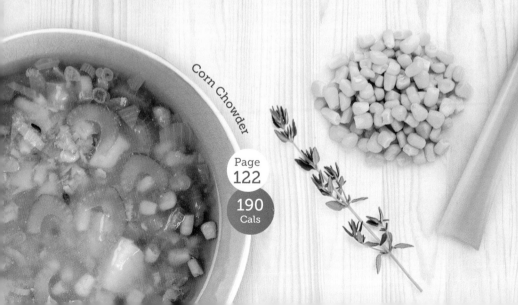

Corn Chowder

Page
122

190
Cals

What is the 8-Week Blood Sugar Diet?

The 8-Week Blood Sugar Diet is an 800 calorie a day eating plan that uses food rather than formulated meal replacement drinks. Its approach describes a Mediterranean, low-carb style of eating. You are encouraged to eat good quality, high-protein foods such as lean meats and fish, low glycaemic index (GI) carb foods such as beans and lentils, a variety of different fruit and low-starch vegetables, full fat dairy products and yogurts, and to choose healthy fats rather than adopt a low-fat approach. The priority of nutritional quality and a plant-based, nutrient dense way of eating differs from more traditional liquid-based, very low-calorie diets.

Chickpea Patties

Page
90

355
Cals

The current advice amongst many health professionals is to follow a diet that encourages a slow, steady weight loss. However, this way of thinking is changing. Everyone has individual needs and consequently no single diet is going to work for all people. An 800 calorie diet can give you a great kick-start and may be more motivating than slower weight loss approaches. The metabolic effects within the body are also likely to be far more rapid, particularly as you reduce the fat stored in your liver and pancreas.

Page
91

355
Cals

What happens after this short period of rapid weight loss and how can you avoid weight re-gain? You need a plan B! After completing your 8 weeks you can incorporate the Mediterranean style of eating into the 5:2 diet or a daily calorie restriction of around 1200-1500 calories per day.

Tuna & Roasted Veg

What are the health benefits of following a very low-calorie diet?

Obesity is linked directly to type 2 diabetes, cancer, high blood pressure, fatty liver disease, heart disease and stroke. It affects mental health and consequently the NHS and the National Institute for Clinical Excellence (NICE) recommend very low-calorie diets as one of a range of weight loss options. As already described on the previous pages, there is promising evidence supporting the use of a very low-calorie diet to reverse abnormally high blood sugar levels, but why a Mediterranean style of eating? Scientific evidence supports the link between a Mediterranean diet and a reduced risk of heart disease, diabetes and certain cancers (such as breast cancer). This is thought to be due to the antioxidant rich foods eaten, such as fruit and vegetables, nuts and seeds.

If you are above your target weight and you do not have a high risk of developing type 2 diabetes, this weight loss approach can still be used. The high-protein, low-carb principles should satisfy your appetite and minimise those hunger pangs all too frequently experienced when dieting.

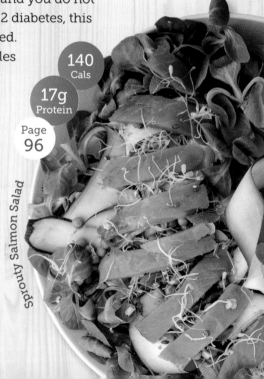

140 Cals

17g Protein

Page 96

Sprouty Salmon Salad

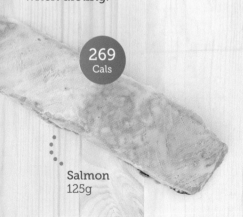

269 Cals

Salmon 125g

Can anyone follow a very low-calorie diet?

If you are considering a very low-calorie diet you should talk to your GP; especially if you are taking medication for diabetes (including insulin) and/or other conditions such as high blood pressure, so they can advise on reducing your medication. If you have diabetes, then commencing a carb-restricted diet whilst continuing your usual insulin dose and/or anti-diabetes medication (such as sulphonylureas) will significantly increase the likelihood of hypoglycaemia.

There are certain situations or medical conditions where a very low-calorie diet would not be advised:

★ Women who are pregnant or breastfeeding

★ Those who are underweight or have a history of an eating disorder

★ Anyone recovering from surgery

★ People under 18 years of age

★ If you have an unstable heart or cerebrovascular disease

★ Those with acute and chronic renal failure

★ Anyone with severe or end-stage liver disease

★ If you have a psychiatric disorder that may interfere with your ability to follow the diet

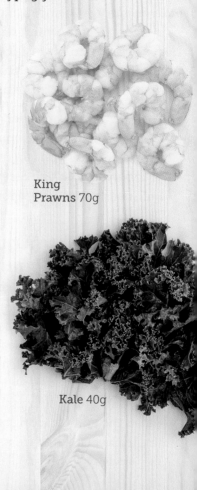

King Prawns 70g

Kale 40g

How to follow a very low-calorie diet

Following a very low-calorie diet means every mouthful has to pack a nutritious and satisfying punch to enable you to stick to it. It requires careful planning to ensure it is balanced and can be incorporated into your daily routine and lifestyle. Due to the restricted intake of nutrients, you may wish to take a daily multivitamin tablet for reassurance.

The following pages offer guidance on which foods to add to your shopping basket and simple changes you can make to ensure your very low-calorie diet is manageable, nutritious and, most importantly, tasty!

Prioritise high quality, lean protein sources

These include lean meat, poultry, fish, eggs, cheese, pulses, nuts and seeds. Lean protein sources should be prioritised with every meal. Protein is essential for the repair and growth of new cells and is known to aid with satiety (feeling of fullness). Processed meats including bacon should be limited to once or twice a week.

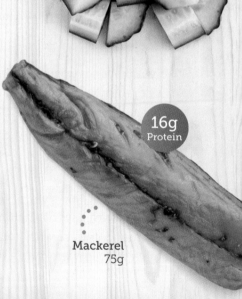

16g
Protein

Mackerel
75g

Leave high GI carbs on the shelf!

Replace high glycaemic index carbs such as white bread, pasta, rice and potatoes with low GI alternatives, for minimal impact on your blood sugar levels. For example, switch rice, bread, white potatoes and breakfast cereals with quinoa, pearl barley, rye bread, jumbo (unprocessed) oats, wild rice and bulgur wheat.

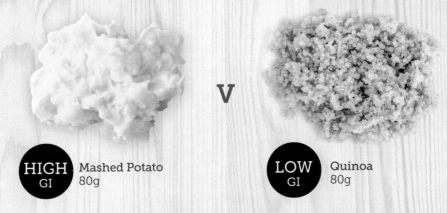

HIGH GI — Mashed Potato 80g

V

LOW GI — Quinoa 80g

Get creative with your carbs!

To minimise swings in your blood sugar levels and keep the calories down, look for alternatives to your usual carbs. For example, replace potato with mashed cannellini beans or parsnip, or replace normal rice with cauliflower rice.

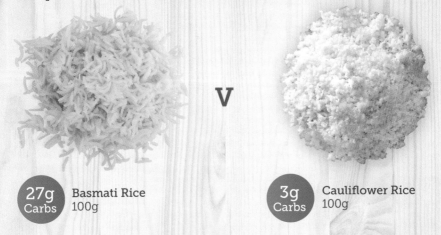

27g Carbs — Basmati Rice 100g

V

3g Carbs — Cauliflower Rice 100g

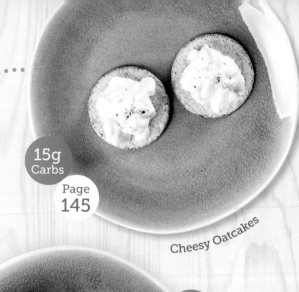

Get savvy with your snacks!

Snack on high-protein, low-carb foods to avoid spikes in your blood sugar levels after eating, which can find you reaching for that extra biscuit! Examples include oatcakes & cottage cheese, celery & nut butter, spicy kale crisps or a small handful of unsalted nuts.

15g Carbs

Page **145**

Cheesy Oatcakes

1g Carbs

Page **136**

Kale Crisps

Almonds
10g

2g Protein

Pistachios
10g

2g Protein

Go nuts for nuts!

The soluble fibre and high-protein content of nuts and seeds will ensure you are kept feeling satisfied between meals with a very minimal impact on your blood sugar levels.

Cashews
10g

2g Protein

Start the day the right way!

Most breakfast products on the market are high in carbs and low in protein, so are therefore unlikely to keep you satisfied until your next meal. Stay fuller for longer with these simple swaps:

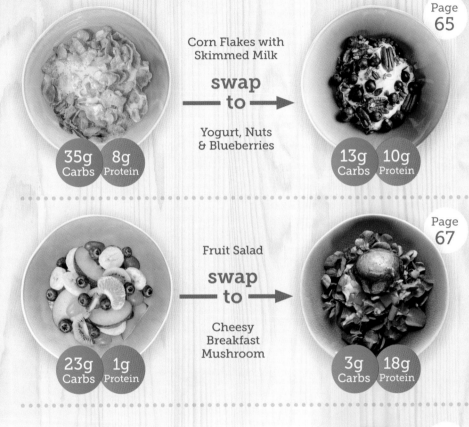

Page
65

Corn Flakes with
Skimmed Milk

swap
to ➔

Yogurt, Nuts
& Blueberries

35g Carbs 8g Protein

13g Carbs 10g Protein

Page
67

Fruit Salad

swap
to ➔

Cheesy
Breakfast
Mushroom

23g Carbs 1g Protein

3g Carbs 18g Protein

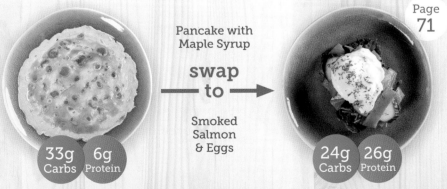

Page
71

Pancake with
Maple Syrup

swap
to ➔

Smoked
Salmon
& Eggs

33g Carbs 6g Protein

24g Carbs 26g Protein

Include lentils and pulses in your meals

They are a great vegetarian protein source, contain slow releasing carbs and are high in soluble fibre; a great combination to keep you feeling full.

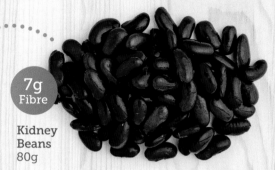

7g
Fibre

Kidney
Beans
80g

Reach for the rainbow!

Vegetables are low in calories and carbs, and are a great source of vitamins and minerals. Using a rainbow of vegetables and fruit in your diet will provide you with a wide variety of nutrients (including vitamins A and C), fibre, phytonutrients and antioxidants, all of which will nourish your body and reduce the risk of health problems.

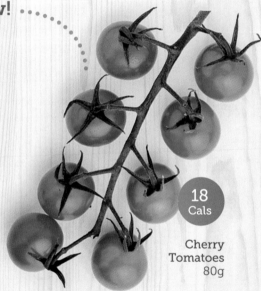

18
Cals

Cherry
Tomatoes
80g

14g
Fat

Avocado
70g

Choose guilt free, healthy fats

Oily fish, olive oil, avocados, nuts and seeds are all high in heart healthy fats and can be included in small portions.

Don't forget to drink up!

The normal recommendation of fluid intake is 1.6 litres for women and 2 litres for men. However, when following a very low-calorie diet, your fluid requirements will be higher, so drink calorie free fluids such as water (with a squeeze of lemon or slice of cucumber) and herbal teas to avoid dehydration and potential side effects such as headaches and constipation.

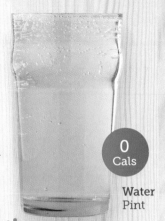

0
Cals

Water
Pint

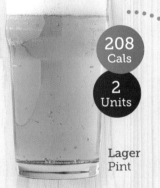

208
Cals

2
Units

Lager
Pint

Avoid alcohol

Alcohol contains a large number of calories and is likely to make you feel more hungry, rather than fill you up.

Limit all sugar and sugary drinks

Latest guidelines are to limit our added sugar intake to 30g per day, to address the increasing obesity and type 2 diabetes epidemic. You can enjoy a small amount of sugar as part of your healthy diet, but choose sugar free options where possible, for example sugar free or diet drinks and squash (which do all contribute towards your fluid intake). Cutting down your sugar intake will help with weight maintenance, weight loss and dental health.

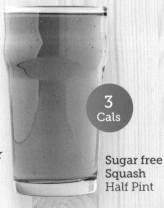

3
Cals

Sugar free
Squash
Half Pint

How to use this book

This book includes 75 carefully-created recipes (plus 20 snacks) for mealtimes across the day, divided into the following sections:

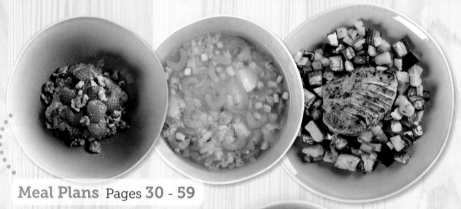

Meal Plans Pages **30 - 59**

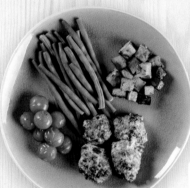

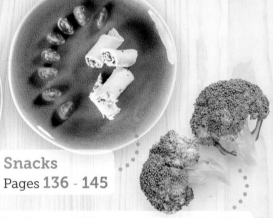

Snacks
Pages **136 - 145**

Recipes
Pages **60 - 135**

Individual Foods Pages **146 - 201**

Within each section, the recipes are listed in calorie order, starting with the lowest calorie recipe. For each dish, the nutritional information for the following nutrients are clearly displayed in colour coded circles:

Cals 5-a-day Fibre SatFat Fat Protein Carbs

Simply browse the variety of recipes and select ones that meet your dietary goal.

Meal Plans

We've devised 30 daily meal plans to offer a range of ideas to suit your individual needs. E.g. brunch and evening meal for a relaxing weekend; two larger meals if you are not a breakfast fan; or breakfast, lunch and an evening meal for those who prefer three meals per day. All daily meal plans contain around 800 calories and different meals can be mixed and matched as long as you keep an eye on the calories. If your daily total comes in at just over the target (e.g. 830 calories), this is okay and you can make it up the next day by choosing a daily plan that comes in just under 800 calories to balance the scales.

There are 15 meal plans with 3 meals per day, and 15 meal plans consisting of 2 meals per day (sometimes including a snack), to suit different lifestyle choices and different dietary requirements, such as a vegetarian diet.

Where the daily plans include snacks, these can be omitted or exchanged for additional food at a mealtime. For example, a handful of nuts as a snack could be replaced with 100g (cooked weight) wild rice with a meal, as they contain a similar amount of calories.

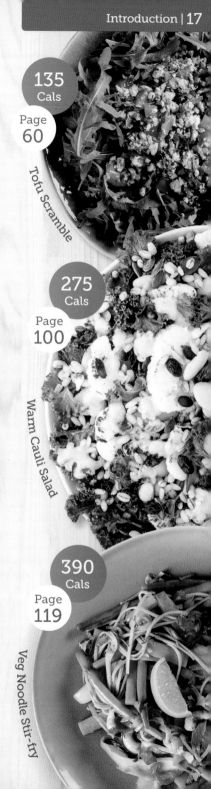

135 Cals
Page 60
Tofu Scramble

275 Cals
Page 100
Warm Cauli Salad

390 Cals
Page 119
Veg Noodle Stir-fry

Recipes

The middle part of the book contains 75 recipes to prepare and enjoy whilst following the diet, ranging from 35-480 calories. Each recipe is for 1 portion but can be doubled up or made into larger quantities and portioned out. Each recipe is simple to make and has been created using the principles of a Mediterranean diet.

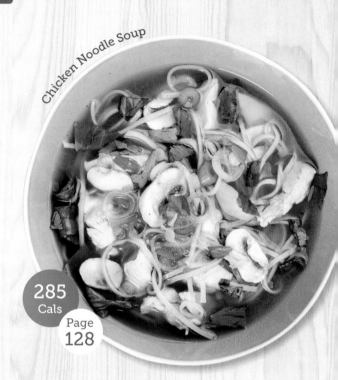

Chicken Noodle Soup

285 Cals

Page **128**

Snacks

Work your way through our 20 healthy and nutritious snack ideas, all under 150 calories. Some even contribute up to 2 of your 5-a-day!

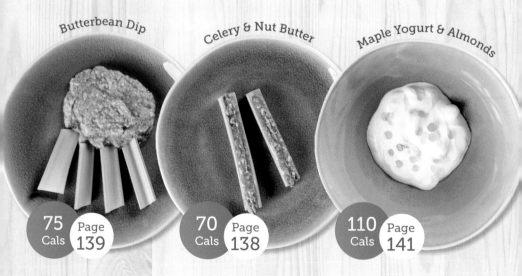

Butterbean Dip

75 Cals

Page **139**

Celery & Nut Butter

70 Cals

Page **138**

Maple Yogurt & Almonds

110 Cals

Page **141**

Individual foods

If you already know your way around the kitchen and have a list of recipes you want to use, then turn to the back of the book for a list of ingredients. The nutritional content of each individual ingredient is shown, giving you the flexibility to build your own recipes. The visual method allows you to quickly select foods in appropriate portions to develop your own 800 calorie meal plans. You may find it useful to write down the details of your creations so you have a record of the nutritional information and can make the recipe again in future.

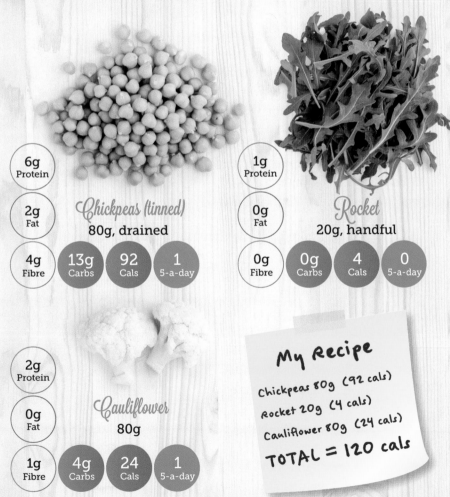

Chickpeas (tinned)
80g, drained

6g Protein
2g Fat
4g Fibre
13g Carbs
92 Cals
1 5-a-day

Rocket
20g, handful

1g Protein
0g Fat
0g Fibre
0g Carbs
4 Cals
0 5-a-day

Cauliflower
80g

2g Protein
0g Fat
1g Fibre
4g Carbs
24 Cals
1 5-a-day

My Recipe

Chickpeas 80g (92 cals)
Rocket 20g (4 cals)
Cauliflower 80g (24 cals)

TOTAL = 120 cals

A few things to note:

★ Planning ahead is key to success. Try to make time each week to write a shopping list and plan for all the meals and snacks you will eat that week.

★ Consider cooking in bulk. This is a great way to always have a meal in the fridge or freezer and to save money. Most of the recipes in this book can be cooked in bulk. A simple way to keep an eye on your calories and portion is to weigh the final dish and then divide into the number of portions you have made.

★ The recipes use average/medium sizes of vegetables and fruit, and weights shown are for the edible part (after being peeled or stoned), unless otherwise stated.

★ Some recipes use a handy measure (e.g. "large handful of watercress") instead of a specific weight. Should you wish to know the exact weight, simply find that portion in the ingredients section. For example, the Quinoa Stuffed Mushrooms recipe on page 81 uses "1 large handful Watercress". Looking at Watercress on page 201, you will see that 1 large handful weighs 20g.

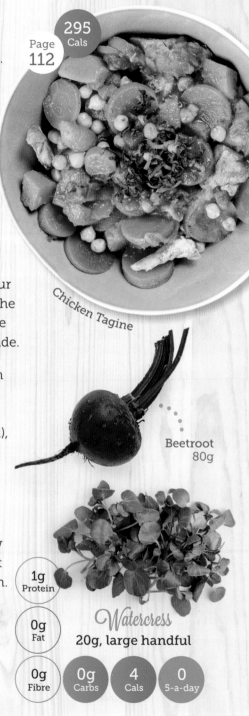

295 Cals

Page 112

Chicken Tagine

Beetroot
80g

1g Protein

0g Fat

0g Fibre

Watercress
20g, large handful

0g Carbs

4 Cals

0 5-a-day

1
Cals

★ If you like your dish spicier, or love the flavour of fresh mint, you can be heavy handed and add more to your taste. Adding these herbs and spices will not affect the calorie content.

Rosemary Sprig

★ Not all the recipes include salt & pepper, so adding such seasoning is down to personal preference. Such addition will not affect the calorie content.

★ The recipes use a mix of uncooked and cooked weights for rice, pasta, couscous, quinoa and pearl barley. The table below outlines the simple conversion for uncooked and cooked weights, although please bear in mind that the longer you cook your pasta and rice, the more water it absorbs, which can affect the final weight of the cooked product.

	Uncooked Weight	Cooked Weight
Couscous	35g	80g
Dried Pasta	45g	100g
Pearl Barley	25g	80g
Quinoa	30g	80g
Rice	35g	100g

White Fusilli Pasta 100g

Pearl Barley 80g

Ingredient Health Benefits

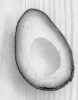

Avocado
A source of potassium; important for regulating blood pressure

Butternut Squash
Protects your immune system, due to its vitamin A content

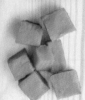

Chickpeas
A source of soluble fibre, important for bowel health and keeping you feeling full

Kale
Power up your immune system with a serving of beta-carotene rich kale

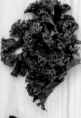

Red Cabbage
High in fibre and water, cabbage helps to prevent constipation

Please note: these benefits must be taken in context of eating a wide variety of foods in your diet and no single ingredient is a 'superfood'.

Broccoli
High in vitamin K, which helps wounds heal properly

Carrots
High in vitamin A, which helps protect eyes and assists with vision in low light

Ginger
Known to alleviate discomfort and pain in the stomach

Pak Choi
Low in calories and fat, so great if you are trying to lose weight

Spinach
Rich in magnesium, to help calm the body and relax muscles

Yellow Pepper
High in beta-carotene (which makes vitamin A) to avoid an itchy scalp and dry hair

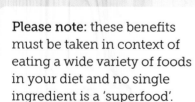

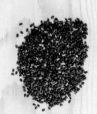

Almonds
Heart healthy and great for skin, due to high vitamin E content

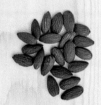

Chia Seeds
A source of omega 3 fatty acids, thought to play a role in preventing dementia

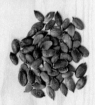

Olive Oil
Rich in monounsaturated fatty acids, shown to have a positive effect on health

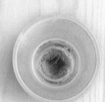

Pumpkin Seeds
A source of magnesium; important for healthy bones and teeth

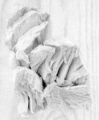

Salmon
High in omega 3 fatty acids which are proven to be protective against heart disease

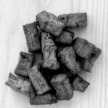

Tofu
Contains all 8 essential amino acids, used by the body to build proteins

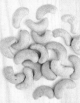

Cashews
Good source of zinc, essential for enhancing memory and thinking skills

Eggs
An eggscellent source of good quality protein, for growth and repair of new cells

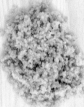

Prawns
A low-calorie source of protein to keep you feeling full

Quinoa
Vegan and gluten free source of good quality protein and magnesium

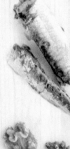

Sardines
High in vitamin D, beneficial to keep bones healthy

Walnuts
Anti-inflammatory, so great for those suffering with joint pain and arthritis

Buying ingredients

★ It is best to use wholegrain pasta and rice to boost fibre content.

★ Use olive oil where possible. Alternatives include rapeseed and groundnut (peanut) oil.

★ Where possible, use fresh, ripe fruit & vegetables.

★ Use good quality, organic produce as often as possible.

★ To keep the cost down, choose vegetables and fruit that are in season. Alternatively, you can replace one vegetable with another that is in season, but be mindful this may change the nutritional content.

★ The thickness of shop bought tahini paste can vary, so you may wish to add more water to achieve the desired consistency.

★ A great way to add variety to your diet and ensure you always have your ingredients to hand is to order a fruit and vegetable box. Each delivery is different so you will receive a variety of different ingredients!

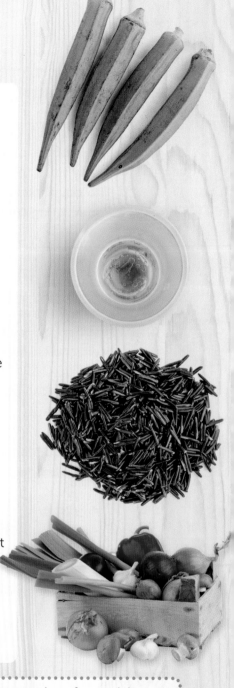

To see our recommended veg box companies, please visit:
www.carbsandcals.com/vegbox

Cooking Glossary

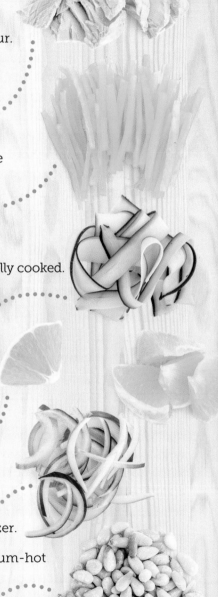

Blanch: Briefly cook vegetables in boiling water to seal in flavour and colour.

Drizzle: Pour a small amount of liquid (e.g. dressing) onto food item or salad.

Flake: Use a fork, or hand, to break cooked fish into smaller pieces and to check if the fish is cooked. If cooked, the fish flesh should fall away easily.

Matchstick: Cut into thin strips.

Mince: Chop very finely.

Parboil: Boil ingredient until it is partially cooked.

Ribbon: Shave vegetables into ribbons using a peeler. If you have a spiralizer, this would work just as well.

Sauté: From the French verb, sauter, meaning 'to jump'. Sautéed food is cooked in a small amount of fat in an open pan on a high heat.

Segment: Divide citrus fruit into smaller sections.

Thinly slice: Slice ingredient into thin slices using a sharp knife or spiralizer.

Toasted nuts: Nuts heated in a medium-hot frying pan (without the addition of oil) to bring out the richness and flavour. Toast for a couple of minutes until fragrant, or light brown in colour.

What next?

Fantastic! You completed the first 8-12 weeks of your weight loss journey and have hopefully achieved your goal. You love seeing your weight go down and the health benefits this brings, and are motivated to continue losing weight. As already explained, a very low-calorie diet should only be followed for 8-12 weeks, as owing to the calorie restriction it is not nutritionally balanced. The core goal with a very low-calorie diet is rapid weight loss and fat loss from the liver and pancreas. The next phase is continuing to follow the dietary principles of a Mediterranean diet (with adequate nutrients including protein, vitamins and minerals), with a greater calorie allowance and even the occasional indulgence.

Calorie restriction is still fundamental for continued weight loss but how you achieve this is up to you. There are many different "miracle" diets popularised by the media that promise health benefits with quick weight loss results. Some diets are considered nutritionally unbalanced (with little or no evidence supporting their sensational health claims). They often advocate cutting out whole food groups entirely, which is unnecessary and potentially dangerous, and therefore do not provide all the nutrients your body requires.

Two nutritionally balanced dietary options include the 5:2 diet or a daily low-calorie diet of 1200-1600 calories. If you prefer to fast (500-600 calories) for 2 days per week and eat 'normally' for the remaining 5 days, then the 5:2 diet may be for you. Or if a higher daily calorie allowance sounds more appealing, then you may wish to plan out meals with a calorie goal per day to aim for.

Thai Vegan Salad

Page
107

390
Cals

Page
128

285
Cals

Chicken Noodle Soup

Making a 5:2 diet meal plan

Using a 5:2 approach to dieting allows many people to achieve weight loss without the feeling of constant deprivation. Similar to the 800 calorie diet, each meal on a fasting day needs to be nutrient rich, tickle your taste buds and keep you feeling full.

How to devise a fasting day meal plan:

1. Decide how you would like to split your calorie allowance for the day. For example, your 500 calories could be made up of two or three meals, spread throughout the day:
   ★ 300 cals for brunch
   ★ 200 cals for dinner

2. Browse the book and decide which meals you enjoyed whilst on the 800 calorie diet and which ones kept you feeling full for the longest. If you noticed you got hungry mid-afternoon, you may want to have a high-protein salad at lunch to keep you feeling satisfied and energised through the afternoon. Alternatively, you may prefer a small light meal at lunch to allow for a larger evening meal.

3. Use this book alongside our 5:2 Diet Photos book for more enjoyable recipes and guidance, to make your fasting days feel like a feast, not a famine!

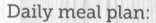

Daily meal plan:

Brunch:
Smoked Salmon & Eggs

290 Cals

26g Protein

Dinner:
Prawn & Avocado Salad

230 Cals

3 5-a-day

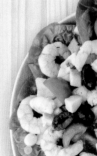

Total: **520** Cals

Making a 1200-1600 calorie meal plan

Following a 1200-1600 calorie diet plan can help you lose around ½kg-1kg (1-2lb) a week (more if you have lots to lose), without feeling that you are depriving yourself of everything. A Mediterranean style of eating ensures you continue to enjoy a healthy, nutritious and satisfying diet, while still achieving weight loss. You can choose how low you want to go. For example, for a gentle approach aim for 1600 calories per day, or if you are keen to continue losing weight at a quicker rate then aim for 1200 calories initially, moving to 1600 calories at a later stage.

Example daily plan:

★ **Breakfast:**
Yogurt, Nuts & Blueberries
(*230 cals, 15g protein*)

★ **Lunch:**
Tuscan Tomato Soup
(*270 cals*), 2 slices rye
bread (*110 cals*) & medium
cappuccino (*116 cals*)

★ **Dinner:**
Thai Green Prawn
Curry (*280 cals*) with
200g (cooked weight)
brown rice (*264 cals*)

Total: 1,270 cals

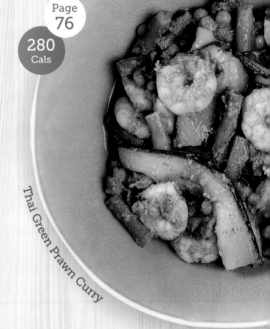

Page
76

280
Cals

Thai Green Prawn Curry

Use this book alongside our SALADS, SMOOTHIES and SOUPS books for more inspiration with meal ideas, and to help you stick to your dietary goal.

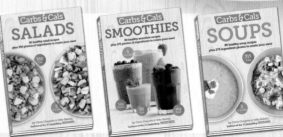

Physical Activity

Finally, incorporating physical activity into your daily routine is important for health and continued weight loss. Physical activity reduces insulin resistance and improves insulin sensitivity, both of which play a role in abnormal blood sugar levels. The current guidelines for exercise in adults are:

★ At least 150 minutes of moderate aerobic activity such as cycling or fast walking every week (e.g. 30 minutes, 5 days a week), AND

★ Strength exercises - two or more days a week. Working all the major muscles (legs, hips, back, abdomen, chest, shoulders and arms).

OR

★ 75 minutes of vigorous aerobic activity, such as running or a game of singles tennis every week, AND

★ Strength exercises - two or more days a week. Working all the major muscles (legs, hips, back, abdomen, chest, shoulders and arms).

OR

★ A mix of moderate and vigorous aerobic activity every week. For example, two 30-minute runs plus 30 minutes of fast walking equates to 150 minutes of moderate aerobic activity, AND

★ Strength exercises - two or more days a week. Working all the major muscles (legs, hips, back, abdomen, chest, shoulders and arms).

There is evidence to show that simply sitting down for long periods is harmful to our health, irrespective of how much exercise is taken. Studies have linked prolonged sitting with type 2 diabetes, heart disease and premature death and so the advice is to move more and sit less! Simple tips to keep you on your feet more include standing or walking while on the phone, using the stairs where possible, doing most types of housework (yes you read that right!) and taking up active hobbies such as gardening.

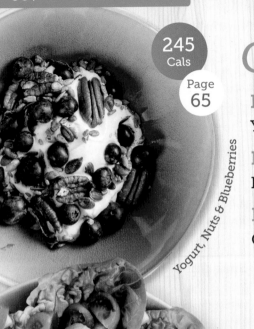

245 Cals

Page **65**

Meal Plan 1

Breakfast
Yogurt, Nuts & Blueberries

Lunch
Prawn & Avocado Salad

Dinner
Okra & Lentil Curry

Yogurt, Nuts & Blueberries

Okra & Lentil Curry

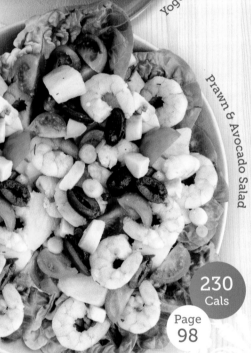

Prawn & Avocado Salad

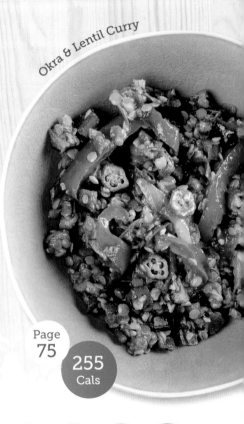

230 Cals

Page **98**

Page **75**

255 Cals

Daily Plan Total:

730 Cals

7½ 5-a-day

20g Fibre

9g SatFat

38g Fat

43g Protein

54g Carbs

Meal Plan 2

Breakfast
Smoked Salmon & Egg

Lunch
Carrot & Lentil Soup

Dinner
Quinoa Stuffed Mushrooms

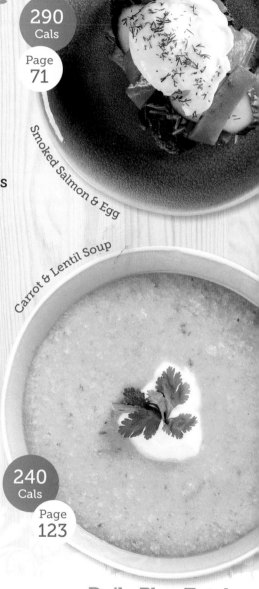

290
Cals

Page
71

Smoked Salmon & Egg

Carrot & Lentil Soup

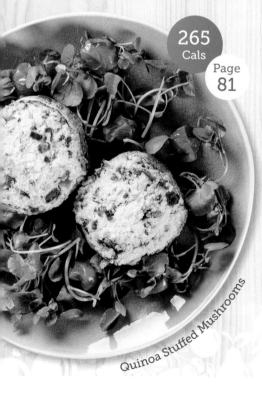

265
Cals

Page
81

240
Cals

Page
123

Quinoa Stuffed Mushrooms

81g
Carbs

50g
Protein

32g
Fat

9g
SatFat

20g
Fibre

Daily Plan Total:

6½
5-a-day

795
Cals

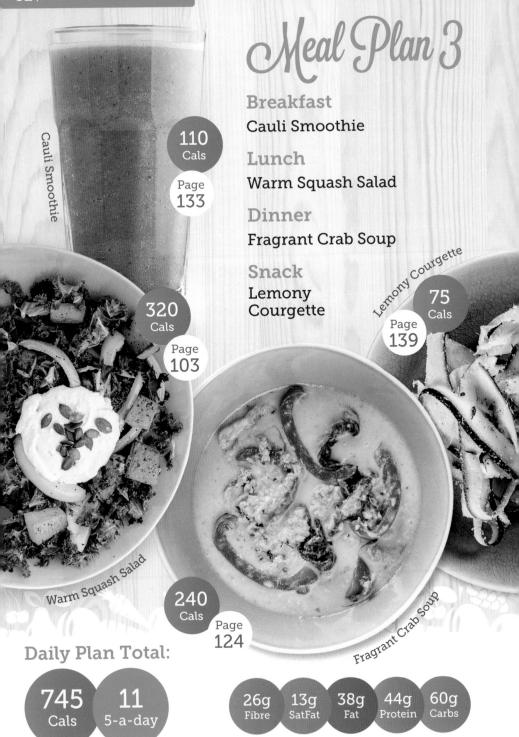

Meal Plan 3

Breakfast
Cauli Smoothie

Lunch
Warm Squash Salad

Dinner
Fragrant Crab Soup

Snack
Lemony Courgette

Cauli Smoothie

110 Cals

Page 133

320 Cals

Page 103

75 Cals

Page 139

Lemony Courgette

Warm Squash Salad

240 Cals

Page 124

Fragrant Crab Soup

Daily Plan Total:

745 Cals

11 5-a-day

26g Fibre

13g SatFat

38g Fat

44g Protein

60g Carbs

Meal Plan 4

245 Cals

Page 66

Chia Seed Breakfast Pot

Breakfast
Chia Seed Breakfast Pot

Lunch
Sprouty Salmon Salad

Dinner
Chicken & Cashew Stir-fry

Snack
Kale Crisps

Sprouty Salmon Salad

Page 136

55 Cals

140 Cals **Page 96**

360 Cals **Page 118**

Kale Crisps

Chicken & Cashew Stir Fry

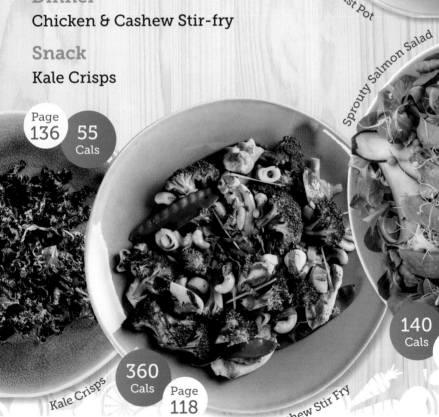

Daily Plan Total:

39g Carbs	78g Protein	36g Fat	7g SatFat	25g Fibre

6 5-a-day   **800 Cals**

Meal Plan 5

200 Cals

Page 61

Breakfast
Egg & Spinach on Rye

Lunch
Black Bean Soup

Dinner
Cheesy Cod Fillets

Egg & Spinach on Rye

Black Bean Soup

325 Cals

Page 84

255 Cals

Page 125

Cheesy Cod Fillets

Daily Plan Total:

780 Cals

6 5-a-day

| 25g Fibre | 11g SatFat | 36g Fat | 60g Protein | 54g Carbs |

Meal Plan 6

Breakfast
Quinoa & Almond Porridge

Lunch
Corn Chowder

Dinner
Tuna & Roasted Veg

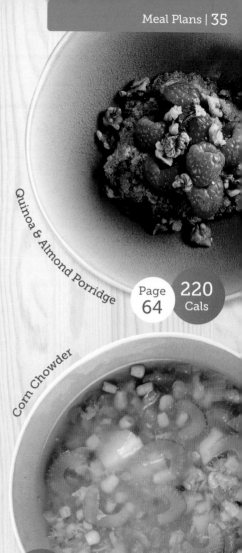

Quinoa & Almond Porridge

Page **64**
220 Cals

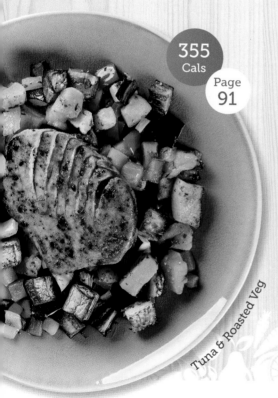

355 Cals
Page **91**

Corn Chowder

Tuna & Roasted Veg

190 Cals
Page **122**

Daily Plan Total:

89g Carbs	55g Protein	24g Fat	3g SatFat	24g Fibre

7½ 5-a-day **765** Cals

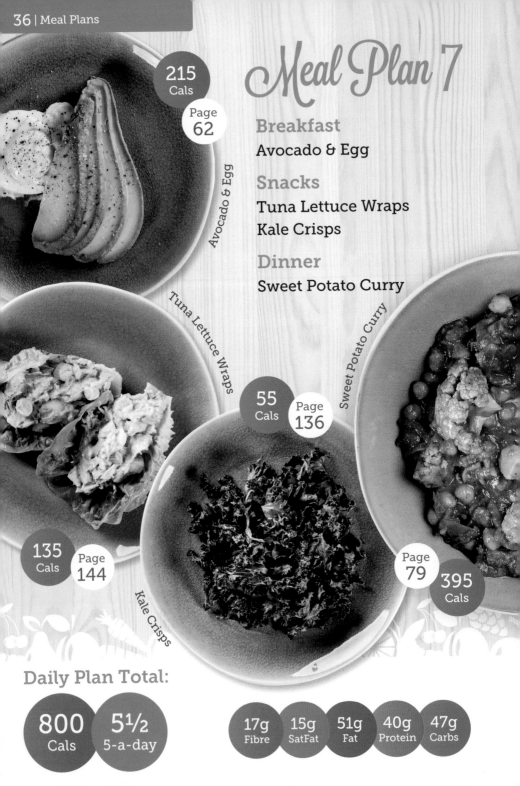

Meal Plan 7

215 Cals
Page 62

Avocado & Egg

Breakfast
Avocado & Egg

Snacks
Tuna Lettuce Wraps
Kale Crisps

Dinner
Sweet Potato Curry

Tuna Lettuce Wraps

Sweet Potato Curry

55 Cals
Page 136

135 Cals
Page 144

Kale Crisps

Page 79
395 Cals

Daily Plan Total:

800 Cals **5½ 5-a-day**

17g Fibre **15g SatFat** **51g Fat** **40g Protein** **47g Carbs**

Meal Plan 8

Breakfast
Carrot Classic Smoothie

Snack
Celery & Nut Butter

Lunch
Mustard Chicken Salad

Dinner
Fish Pie

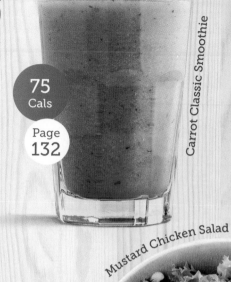

Carrot Classic Smoothie

75 Cals

Page **132**

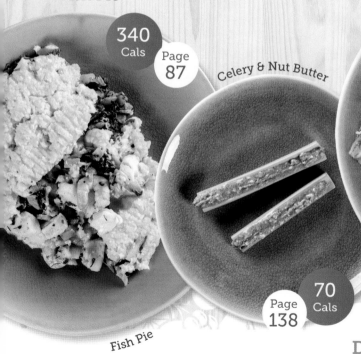

340 Cals

Page **87**

Mustard Chicken Salad

Celery & Nut Butter

70 Cals

Page **138**

Page **102**

305 Cals

Fish Pie

59g Carbs	70g Protein	30g Fat	8g SatFat	21g Fibre

Daily Plan Total:

10½ 5-a-day   **790** Cals

Meal Plan 9

135 Cals

Page 60

Tofu Scramble

Breakfast
Tofu Scramble

Lunch
Warm Cauli Salad

Dinner
Veg Noodle Stir-fry

Warm Cauli Salad

390 Cals

Page 119

275 Cals

Page 100

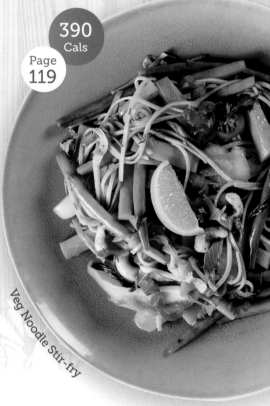

Veg Noodle Stir-fry

Daily Plan Total:

800 Cals

8 5-a-day

23g Fibre

5g SatFat

33g Fat

36g Protein

92g Carbs

Meal Plan 10

Breakfast
Fruity Porridge

Lunch
Tom Yum Soup

Dinner
Chicken Tagine

Snack
Nectarine

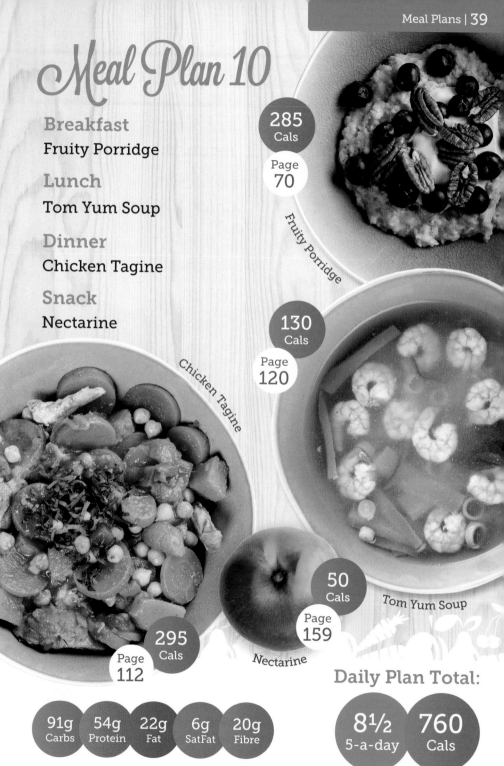

285 Cals
Page 70
Fruity Porridge

130 Cals
Page 120
Chicken Tagine

295 Cals
Page 112

50 Cals
Page 159
Nectarine

Tom Yum Soup

Daily Plan Total:

91g Carbs | 54g Protein | 22g Fat | 6g SatFat | 20g Fibre

8½ 5-a-day | 760 Cals

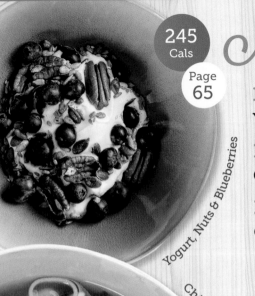

245 Cals

Page **65**

Meal Plan 11

Breakfast
Yogurt, Nuts & Blueberries

Lunch
Chicken Noodle Soup

Dinner
Cauliflower Risotto

Yogurt, Nuts & Blueberries

Chicken Noodle Soup

Cauliflower Risotto

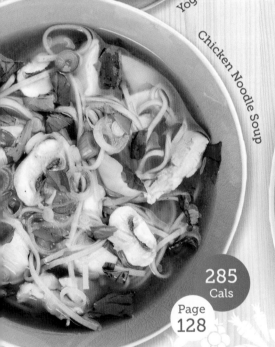

265 Cals

Page **80**

285 Cals

Page **128**

Daily Plan Total:

795 Cals

5 5-a-day

14g Fibre

12g SatFat

34g Fat

54g Protein

70g Carbs

Meal Plan 12

Breakfast
Avocado & Egg

Lunch
Olive Steak Salad

Dinner
Jamaican Chicken Curry

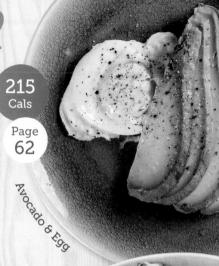

215 Cals

Page 62

Avocado & Egg

360 Cals

Page 77

Olive Steak Salad

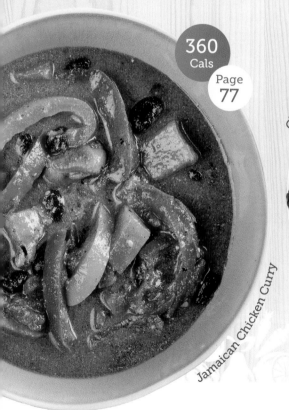

Page 97

225 Cals

Jamaican Chicken Curry

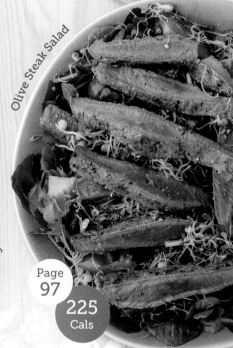

40g Carbs | 71g Protein | 41g Fat | 10g SatFat | 20g Fibre

Daily Plan Total:

7 5-a-day | 800 Cals

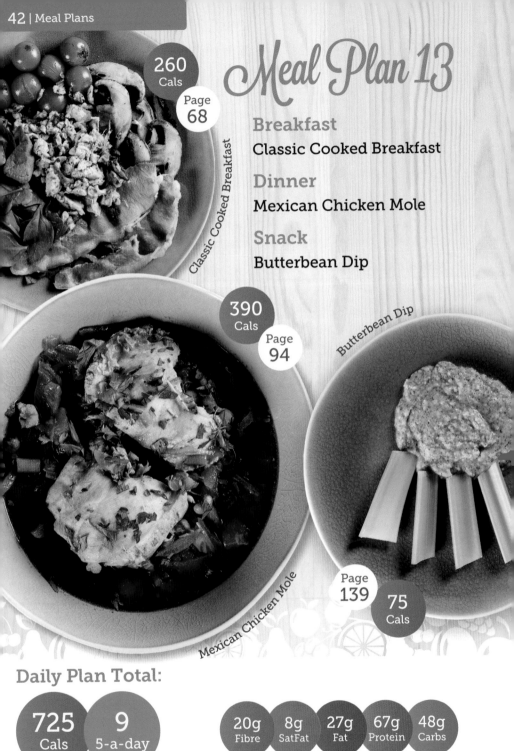

Meal Plan 13

260
Cals

Page **68**

Classic Cooked Breakfast

Breakfast
Classic Cooked Breakfast

Dinner
Mexican Chicken Mole

Snack
Butterbean Dip

390
Cals

Page **94**

Butterbean Dip

Mexican Chicken Mole

Page **139**

75
Cals

Daily Plan Total:

725
Cals

9
5-a-day

20g
Fibre

8g
SatFat

27g
Fat

67g
Protein

48g
Carbs

Meal Plan 14

Breakfast
Wild Rice Kedgeree

Dinner
Lamb & Rosemary Stew

Snack
Turkey Rolls

315 Cals

Page 74

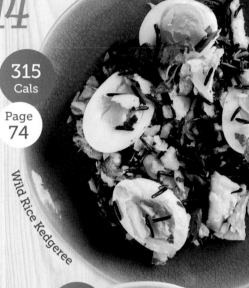

Wild Rice Kedgeree

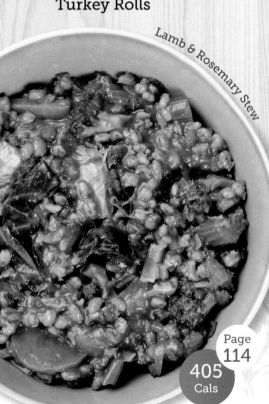

Lamb & Rosemary Stew

65 Cals

Page 137

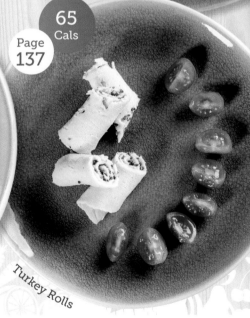

Turkey Rolls

Page 114
405 Cals

Daily Plan Total:

68g Carbs   65g Protein   25g Fat   8g SatFat   15g Fibre

3½ 5-a-day   785 Cals

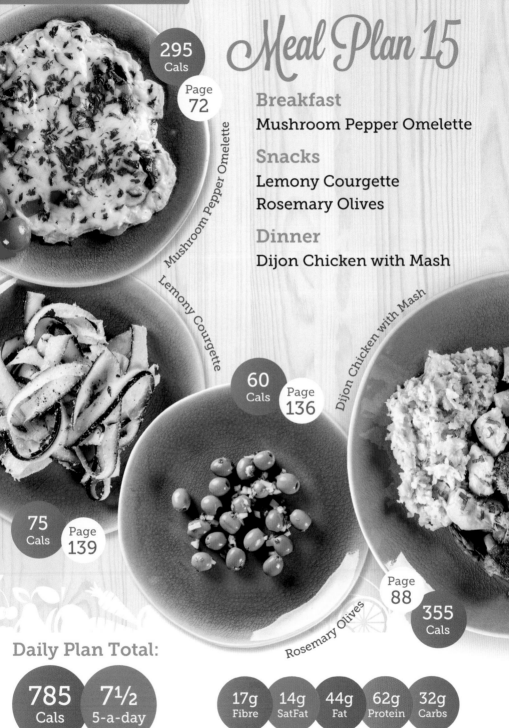

Meal Plan 15

295 Cals

Page 72

Breakfast
Mushroom Pepper Omelette

Snacks
Lemony Courgette
Rosemary Olives

Dinner
Dijon Chicken with Mash

Mushroom Pepper Omelette

Lemony Courgette

Dijon Chicken with Mash

60 Cals

Page 136

75 Cals

Page 139

Page 88

355 Cals

Rosemary Olives

Daily Plan Total:

785 Cals

7½ 5-a-day

17g Fibre

14g SatFat

44g Fat

62g Protein

32g Carbs

Meal Plan 16

Breakfast
Veggie Breakfast

Snacks
Roasted Pumpkin Seeds
Raspberries

Dinner
Tofu & Bean Stir-fry

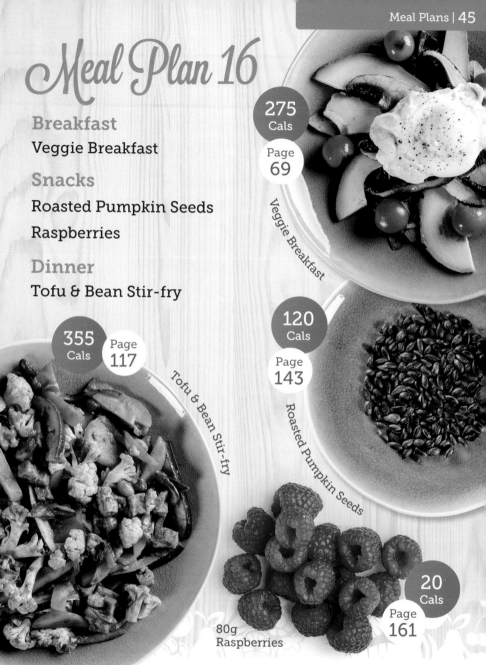

275 Cals — Page 69

Veggie Breakfast

120 Cals — Page 143

Roasted Pumpkin Seeds

355 Cals — Page 117

Tofu & Bean Stir-fry

20 Cals — Page 161

80g Raspberries

Daily Plan Total:

36g Carbs	44g Protein	50g Fat	10g SatFat	18g Fibre

8 5-a-day | **770** Cals

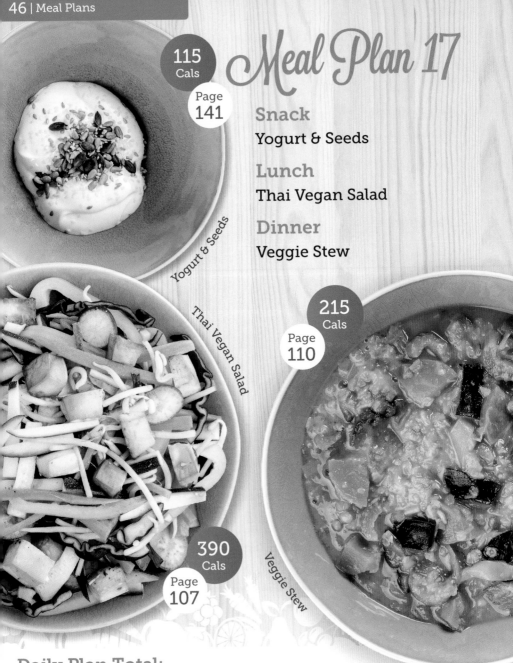

Meal Plan 17

115 Cals

Page **141**

Snack
Yogurt & Seeds

Lunch
Thai Vegan Salad

Dinner
Veggie Stew

Yogurt & Seeds

Thai Vegan Salad

215 Cals

Page **110**

390 Cals

Page **107**

Veggie Stew

Daily Plan Total:

720 Cals

10½ 5-a-day

25g Fibre

6g SatFat

34g Fat

38g Protein

69g Carbs

Meal Plan 18

Breakfast
Tofu Scramble

Snack
Celery & Nut Butter

Drink
Medium Cappuccino (whole)

Dinner
Roots & Lentil Salad

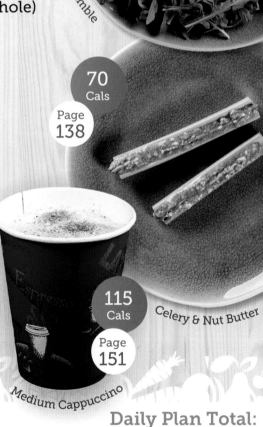

135
Cals

Page
60

Tofu Scramble

70
Cals

Page
138

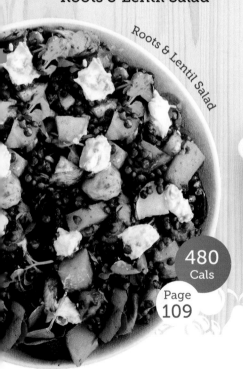

Roots & Lentil Salad

480
Cals

Page
109

115
Cals

Page
151

Medium Cappuccino

Celery & Nut Butter

Daily Plan Total:

76g Carbs	44g Protein	35g Fat	10g SatFat	23g Fibre

8
5-a-day

800
Cals

Meal Plan 19

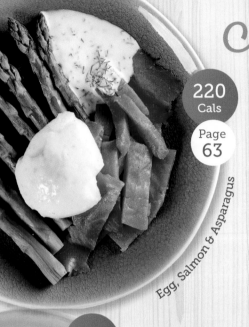

220 Cals

Page **63**

Egg, Salmon & Asparagus

Breakfast
Egg, Salmon & Asparagus

Snacks
Maple Yogurt & Almonds
Spicy Chickpeas

Dinner
Thai Green Prawn Curry

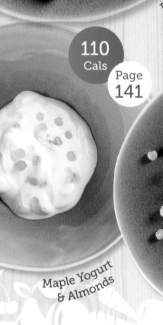

110 Cals

Page **141**

Maple Yogurt & Almonds

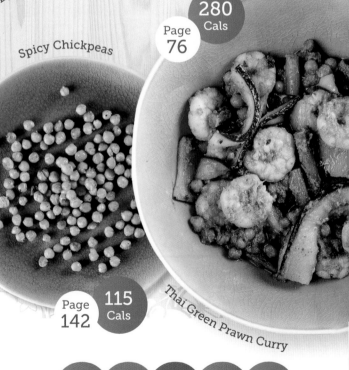

Spicy Chickpeas

280 Cals

Page **76**

Page **142**

115 Cals

Thai Green Prawn Curry

Daily Plan Total:

725 Cals

4 5-a-day

12g Fibre

16g SatFat

40g Fat

58g Protein

35g Carbs

Meal Plan 20

Breakfast
Cheesy Breakfast Mushroom

Lunch
Pick up a Pepper Smoothie

Dinner
Chickpea Patties

Snack
Blackberries

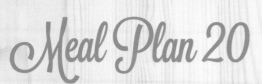

Cheesy Breakfast Mushroom

Page 67 — 250 Cals

125 Cals — Page 134

Chickpea Patties

Pick up a Pepper Smoothie

20 Cals — Page 158

Page 90 — 355 Cals

80g Blackberries

Daily Plan Total:

9 5-a-day — 750 Cals

45g Carbs | 41g Protein | 46g Fat | 16g SatFat | 22g Fibre

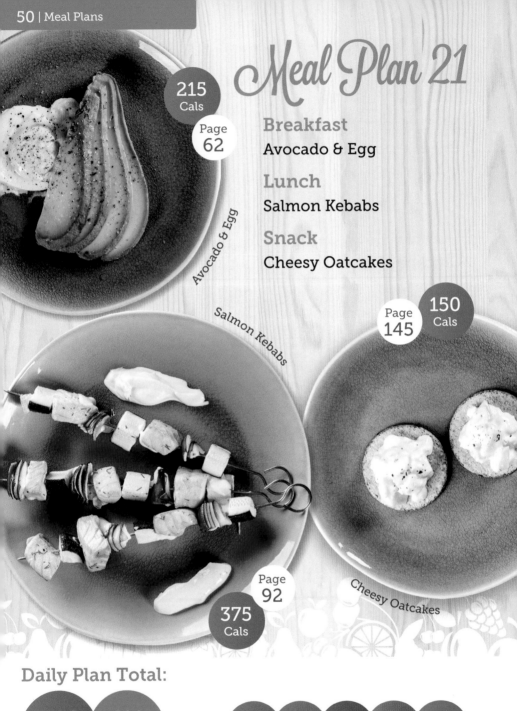

Meal Plan 21

215 Cals

Page 62

Avocado & Egg

Breakfast
Avocado & Egg

Lunch
Salmon Kebabs

Snack
Cheesy Oatcakes

Salmon Kebabs

Page 145

150 Cals

Page 92

375 Cals

Cheesy Oatcakes

Daily Plan Total:

740 Cals

4½ 5-a-day

10g Fibre

12g SatFat

47g Fat

52g Protein

29g Carbs

Meal Plan 22

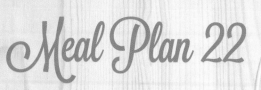

Breakfast
Quinoa & Almond Porridge

Lunch
Grass in a Glass Smoothie

Snack
Tuna Lettuce Wraps

Dinner
Parsnip Cauliflower Soup

Quinoa & Almond Porridge

Page 64 — 220 Cals

270 Cals — Page 127

Tuna Lettuce Wraps

175 Cals — Page 135

Parsnip Cauliflower Soup

135 Cals — Page 144

Grass in a Glass Smoothie

Daily Plan Total:

85g Carbs | 37g Protein | 36g Fat | 5g SatFat | 27g Fibre

6½ 5-a-day | 800 Cals

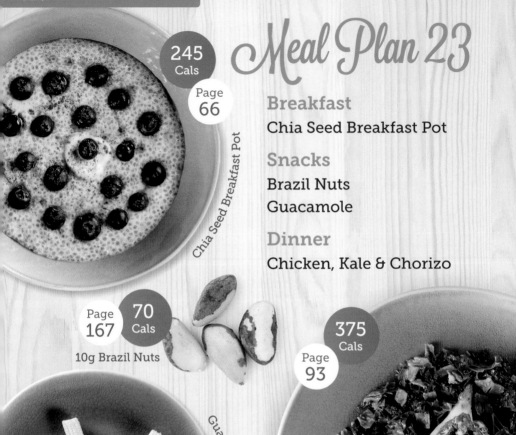

Meal Plan 23

Breakfast
Chia Seed Breakfast Pot

Snacks
Brazil Nuts
Guacamole

Dinner
Chicken, Kale & Chorizo

245
Cals

Page
66

Chia Seed Breakfast Pot

Page
167

70
Cals

10g Brazil Nuts

375
Cals

Page
93

Guacamole

100
Cals

Page
140

Chicken, Kale & Chorizo

Daily Plan Total:

790
Cals

3½
5-a-day

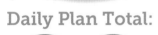

| 19g Fibre | 14g SatFat | 47g Fat | 59g Protein | 29g Carbs |

Meal Plan 24

Snack
Mozzarella & Tomato

Lunch
Beef & Mushroom Stir-fry

Dinner
Asparagus Frittata

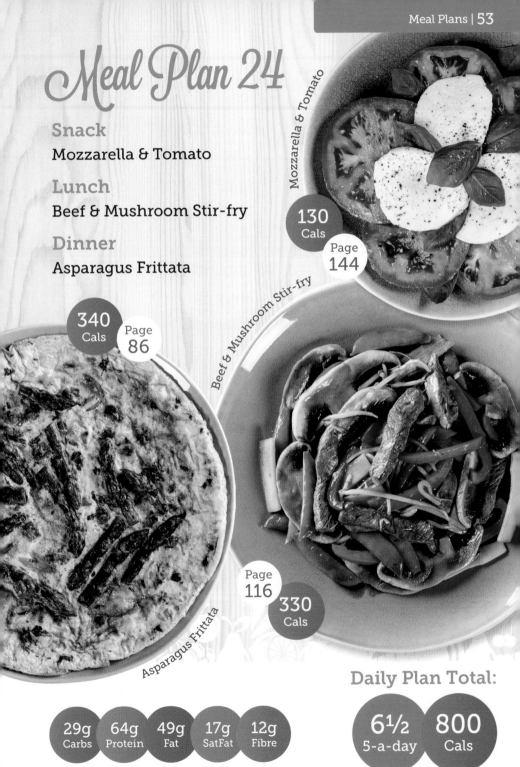

Mozzarella & Tomato

130 Cals

Page 144

Beef & Mushroom Stir-fry

340 Cals

Page 86

Page 116

330 Cals

Asparagus Frittata

Daily Plan Total:

29g Carbs	64g Protein	49g Fat	17g SatFat	12g Fibre

6½ 5-a-day

800 Cals

Meal Plan 25

Breakfast
Egg & Mackerel Salad

Lunch
Carrot & Lentil Soup

Dinner
Hey Pesto! Smoothie

Snack
Mixed Nuts

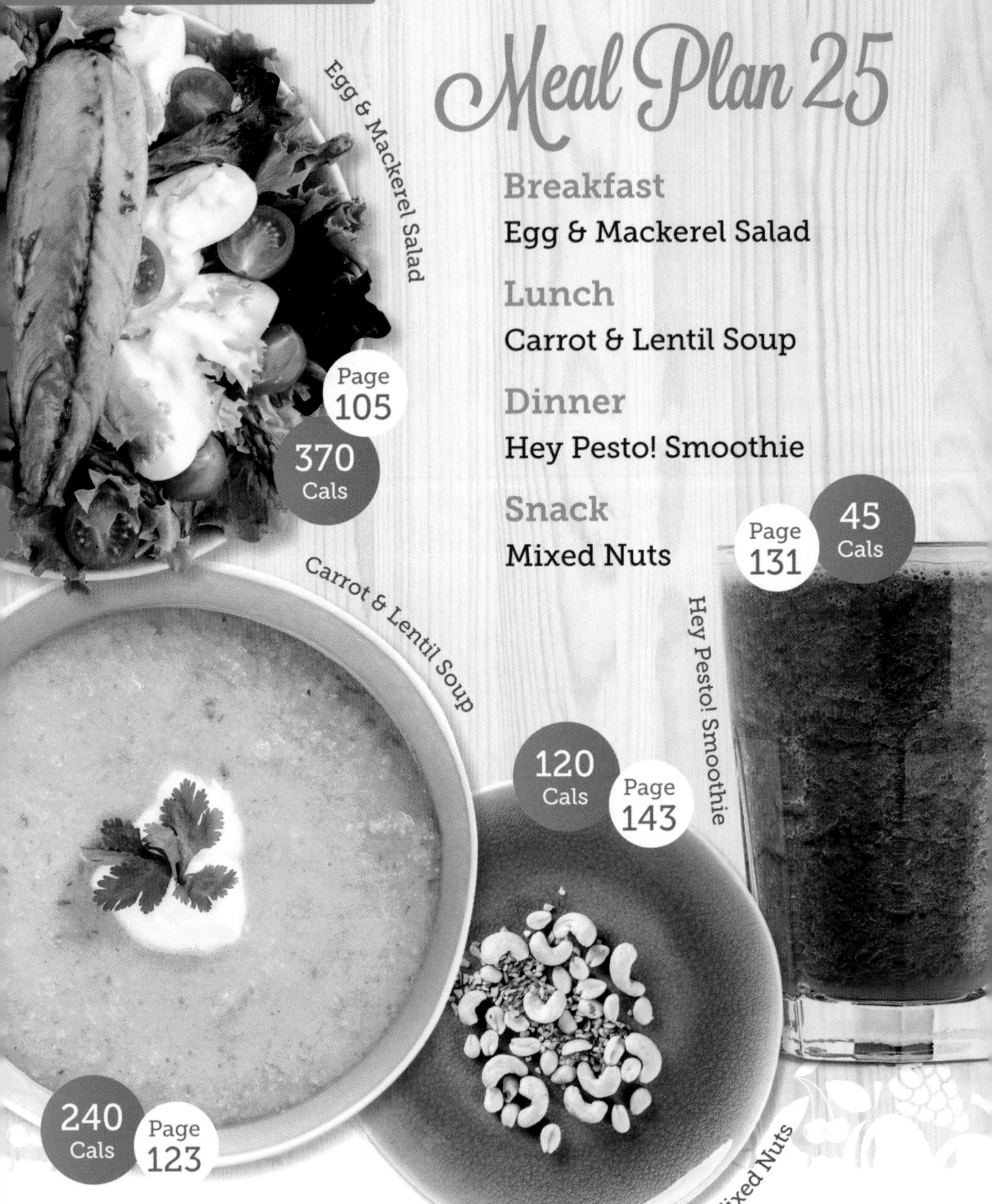

Egg & Mackerel Salad
Page 105
370 Cals

Carrot & Lentil Soup
240 Cals
Page 123

Hey Pesto! Smoothie
Page 131
45 Cals

Mixed Nuts
120 Cals
Page 143

Daily Plan Total:

775 Cals

7½ 5-a-day

17g Fibre

10g SatFat

45g Fat

47g Protein

45g Carbs

Meal Plan 26

Breakfast
Huevos Rancheros

Lunch
Egg & Quinoa Salad

Snack
Olives, Feta & Veg

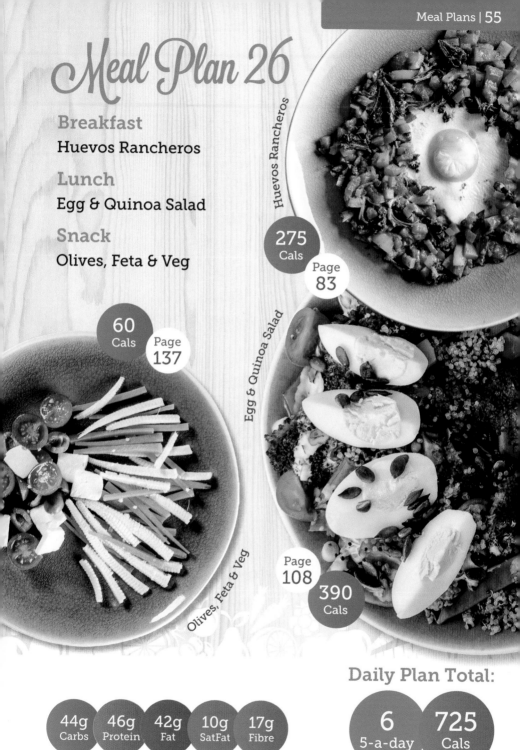

Huevos Rancheros

275 Cals

Page **83**

Egg & Quinoa Salad

60 Cals

Page **137**

Page **108**

390 Cals

Olives, Feta & Veg

Daily Plan Total:

44g Carbs	46g Protein	42g Fat	10g SatFat	17g Fibre

6 5-a-day

725 Cals

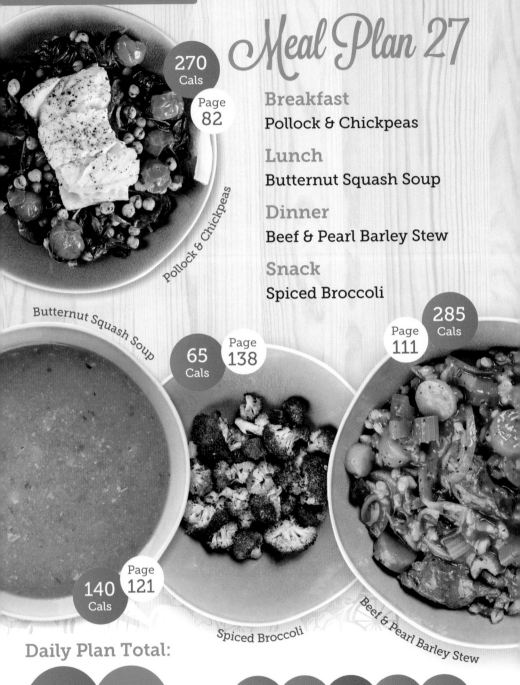

Meal Plan 27

270 Cals
Page **82**

Breakfast
Pollock & Chickpeas

Lunch
Butternut Squash Soup

Dinner
Beef & Pearl Barley Stew

Snack
Spiced Broccoli

Pollock & Chickpeas

Butternut Squash Soup

65 Cals
Page **138**

285 Cals
Page **111**

140 Cals
Page **121**

Spiced Broccoli

Beef & Pearl Barley Stew

Daily Plan Total:

760 Cals **12** 5-a-day

31g Fibre **3g** SatFat **18g** Fat **62g** Protein **91g** Carbs

Meal Plan 28

Snack
Butterbean Dip

Lunch
Moroccan Veg & Chickpeas

Dinner
Sticky Salmon Salad

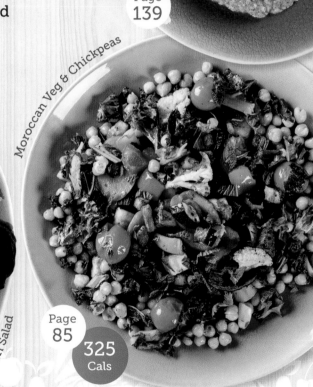

Butterbean Dip

75 Cals

Page **139**

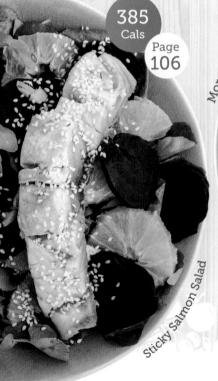

385 Cals

Page **106**

Moroccan Veg & Chickpeas

Sticky Salmon Salad

Page **85**

325 Cals

Daily Plan Total:

64g Carbs	58g Protein	35g Fat	6g SatFat	28g Fibre

11½ 5-a-day | **785** Cals

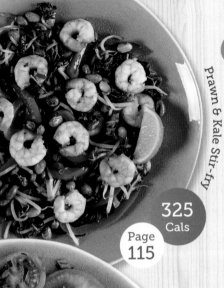

Meal Plan 29

Breakfast
Prawn & Kale Stir-fry

Lunch
Triple Tomato Salad

Dinner
Vegetable & Bean Chilli

Prawn & Kale Stir-fry

325 Cals

Page **115**

Triple Tomato Salad

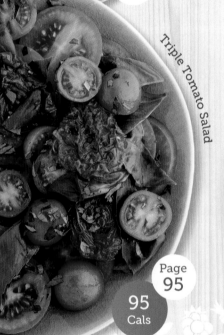

380 Cals

Page **113**

Page **95**

95 Cals

Vegetable & Bean Chilli

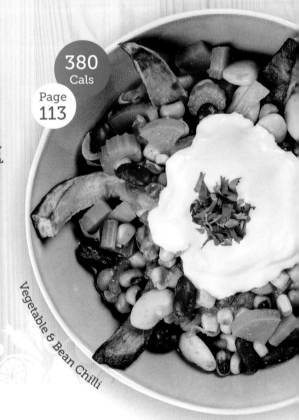

Daily Plan Total:

800 Cals

10½ 5-a-day

31g Fibre

5g SatFat

25g Fat

51g Protein

90g Carbs

Meal Plan 30

Snack
Soya Beans

Lunch
Spring Chicken Soup

Dinner
Lamb Dhansak

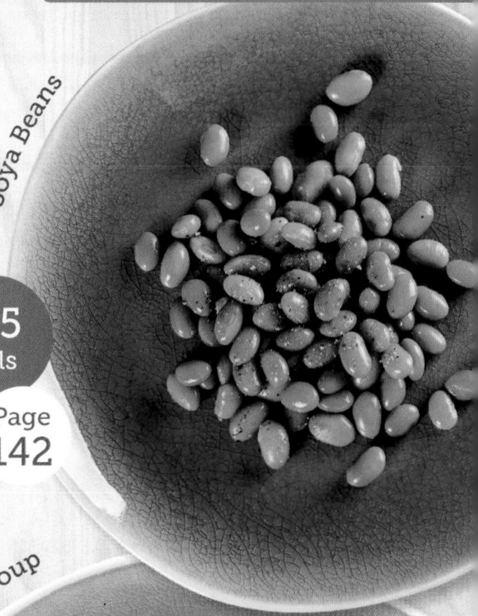

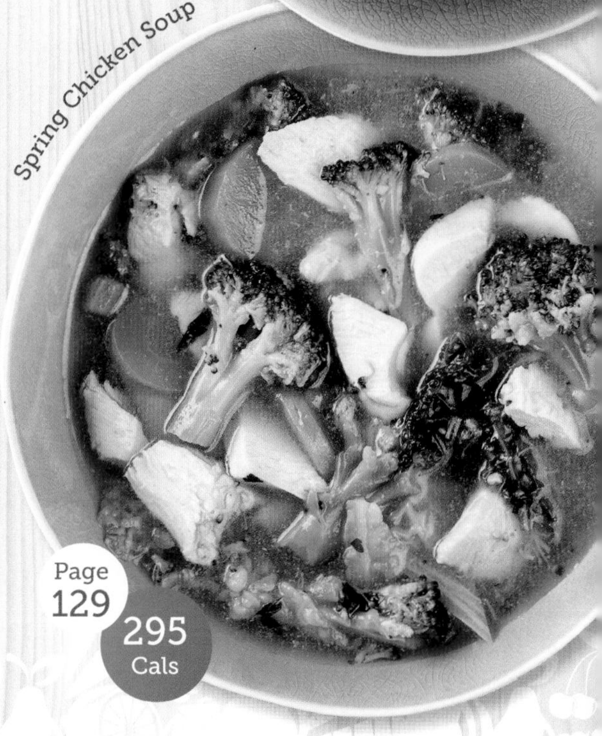

Soya Beans

115
Cals

Page
142

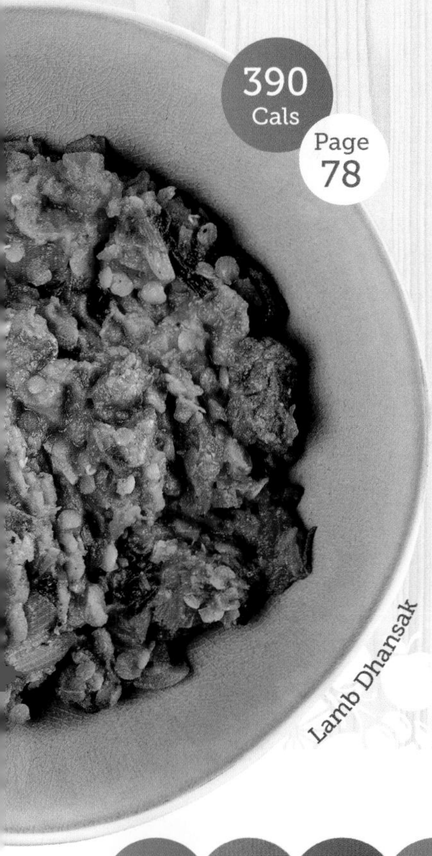

390
Cals

Page
78

Spring Chicken Soup

Page
129

295
Cals

Lamb Dhansak

Daily Plan Total:

59g Carbs	85g Protein	25g Fat	7g SatFat	21g Fibre

7½ 5-a-day | **800** Cals

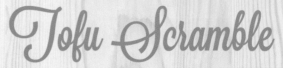

Tofu Scramble

Our lowest-calorie breakfast, with 13g protein and 2 portions of veg - a great start to the day!

Ingredients

8	**Cherry Tomatoes** (quartered)
1/8	**Green Pepper** (diced)
1/8	**Red Pepper** (diced)
1/3	**Red Onion** (finely chopped)
150g	**Silken Tofu** (crumbled)
1 sprig	**Parsley** (large, chopped)
1	handful **Rocket**

Preparation

1. Dry fry the **tomatoes**, **pepper** and **onion** for 5 mins.
2. Add the **tofu** and heat through.
3. Remove from the heat and stir in the **parsley**.
4. Serve on a bed of **rocket**.

135 Cals

2 5-a-day

3g Fibre

1g SatFat

5g Fat

13g Protein

11g Carbs

Weight | 260g

Egg & Spinach on Rye

This quick & easy recipe gives the classic eggs Florentine a low-calorie twist

Ingredients

1	**Egg**
2	handfuls **Spinach**
1 slice	**Rye Bread**

Preparation

1. Poach the **egg** in boiling water (with or without vinegar) for 4 mins.
2. Meanwhile, wilt the **spinach** in a pan with 1 tbsp water for 2 mins, and toast the **bread**.
3. Serve the toast topped with wilted spinach and the egg.

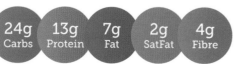

24g Carbs	13g Protein	7g Fat	2g SatFat	4g Fibre

Weight | 140g

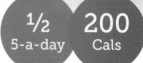

½ 5-a-day	200 Cals

Avocado & Egg

This combination of avo & egg is a great source of good-quality protein & healthy fats

Ingredients

1   **Egg**
¼   **Lemon** (juice only)
½   **Avocado** (sliced)

Preparation

1. Poach the **egg** in boiling water (with or without vinegar) for 4 mins.
2. Drizzle the **lemon juice** over the **avocado** and serve with the poached egg.

215 Cals

1 5-a-day

3g Fibre

4g SatFat

19g Fat

9g Protein

2g Carbs

Weight | 120g

Egg, Salmon & Asparagus

Start your day a colourful way with this smorgasbord of flavours!

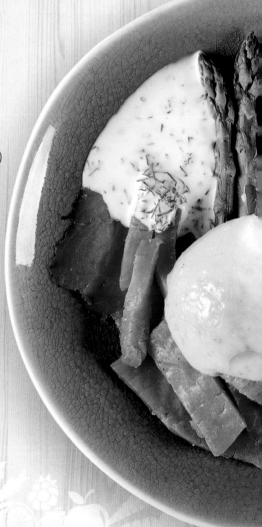

Ingredients
1	**Egg**
40g	**Natural Yogurt**
1 sprig	**Dill** (finely chopped)
¼	**Lemon** (juice only)
50g	**Smoked Salmon**
80g	**Asparagus** (blanched)

Preparation
1. Poach the **egg** in boiling water (with or without vinegar) for 4 mins.
2. To make the dressing, mix the **yogurt**, **dill** and **lemon juice**.
3. Serve the **salmon** and **asparagus** topped with the egg and dressing.

5g Carbs **24g** Protein **12g** Fat **3g** SatFat **2g** Fibre

1 5-a-day **220** Cals

Weight | 255g

Quinoa & Almond Porridge

It's fruity, it's nutty (and also gluten-free!)

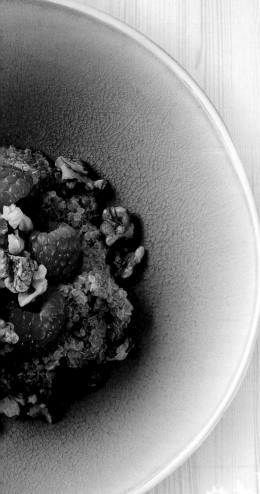

Ingredients

30g	dried **Quinoa**
150ml	**Almond Milk**
½	**Vanilla Pod** (seeds only)
pinch	**Cinnamon** (ground)
8	**Raspberries**
1 tbsp	**Walnuts** (chopped)

Preparation

1. Heat the **quinoa** with the **almond milk**, **vanilla seeds** and **cinnamon**.

2. Bring to the boil and simmer for 15 mins.

3. Spoon into a bowl and top with **raspberries** and **walnuts**.

220 Cals

½ 5-a-day

5g Fibre

1g SatFat

10g Fat

7g Protein

25g Carbs

Weight | 175g

Yogurt, Nuts & Blueberries

A medley of textures... creamy yogurt, crunchy nuts & seeds, and juicy blueberry bombs

Ingredients

1 tbsp	**Pecans** (chopped)
1 tbsp	**Mixed Seeds**
pinch	**Cinnamon** (ground)
150g	**Natural Yogurt**
40g	**Blueberries**

Preparation

1. In a dry pan over a medium heat, toast the **pecans** and **seeds** with **cinnamon** until aromatic.

2. Spoon the **yogurt** into a bowl, and serve topped with the toasted nuts and **blueberries**.

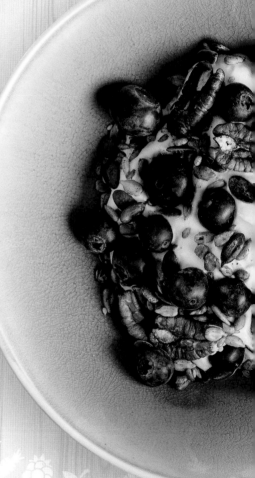

13g Carbs

10g Protein

17g Fat

5g SatFat

3g Fibre

Weight | 205g

1/2 5-a-day

245 Cals

Chia Seed Breakfast Pot

This vanilla-infused brekkie provides a third of your daily fibre needs before you've left the house!

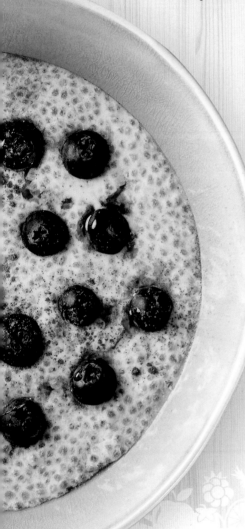

Ingredients

25g	Dark Chia Seeds
180ml	Almond Milk
½	Vanilla Pod (seeds only)
40g	Greek Yogurt
40g	Blueberries
1 tsp	Maple Syrup
pinch	Cinnamon (ground)

Preparation

1. Combine the **chia seeds** with the **almond milk** and **vanilla seeds**.

2. Soak in the fridge for 6 hours, or overnight.

3. Mix the **yogurt** through the chia seeds.

4. Top with **blueberries**, **maple syrup** and a pinch of **cinnamon**.

245 Cals

½ 5-a-day

10g Fibre

3g SatFat

14g Fat

9g Protein

18g Carbs

Weight | 295g

Cheesy Breakfast Mushroom

Mushroom burger for breakfast? Yes please!
This one is flavoured with garlic and cheese

Ingredients

2	**Portobello Mushrooms**
¼	**Red Romano Pepper** (chopped)
1 clove	**Garlic** (minced)
50g	**Smoked Cheddar** (sliced)
1	large handful **Watercress**

Preparation

1. Lay one **mushroom** topside down on a baking tray.
2. Sprinkle with half the **pepper** and half the **garlic**.
3. Lay the sliced **cheese** on top, then the remaining pepper and garlic, to make a stack.
4. Top with the other mushroom and press down gently.
5. Bake for 12 mins at 180°C, turning once.
6. Serve on a bed of **watercress**.

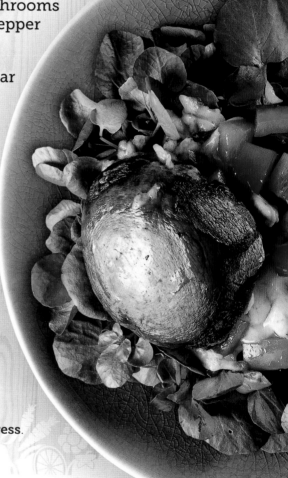

3g	18g	18g	11g	2g
Carbs	Protein	Fat	SatFat	Fibre

Weight | 200g

1½	250
5-a-day	Cals

Classic Cooked Breakfast

If you can't resist a fry-up, try this for only 260 cals!
It's low-carb and has 2 of your 5-a-day

Ingredients

2	**Back Bacon** rashers
80g	**Mushrooms** (sliced)
8	**Cherry Tomatoes** (on the vine)
1	**Egg** (whisked)
1	handful **Spinach**

Preparation

1. Dry fry the **bacon**, **mushrooms** and **tomatoes** for 10 mins.

2. Set aside the mixture on a warm plate, then add the **egg** to the same pan and stir until scrambled.

3. Serve with fresh **spinach** on the side.

260 Cals

2 5-a-day

1g Fibre

5g SatFat

16g Fat

20g Protein

5g Carbs

Weight | 190g

Veggie Breakfast

This vibrant veggie ensemble is loaded with nutrients and 3½ of your 5-a-day

Ingredients

1	**Egg**
80g	**Mushrooms** (sliced)
8	**Cherry Tomatoes** (on the vine)
1 tsp	**Olive Oil**
2	handfuls **Spinach**
½	**Avocado** (sliced)

Preparation

1. Poach the **egg** in boiling water (with or without vinegar) for 4 mins.

2. Meanwhile, pan fry the **mushrooms** and **tomatoes** in 1 tsp **oil**, until they start to colour.

3. Add the **spinach** for a couple of minutes, until it starts to wilt.

4. Serve as a stack, with spinach on the bottom, **avocado**, mushroom and topped with the egg.

5. Finally, decorate the plate with the tomatoes and any juices from the pan.

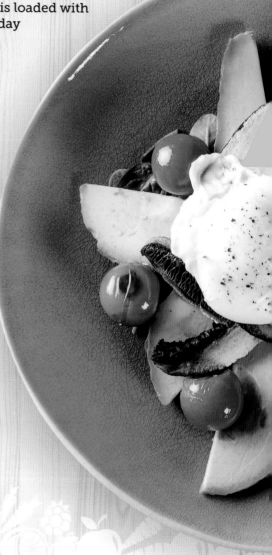

5g Carbs	**12g** Protein	**24g** Fat	**5g** SatFat	**5g** Fibre

Weight | 245g

3½ 5-a-day

275 Cals

Fruity Porridge

Stay full all morning with this tasty
bowl of slow releasing carbs

Ingredients

4 tbsp	Jumbo Oats
150ml	Milk (whole)
¼	Apple (grated)
1 tbsp	Pecans
40g	Blueberries
1 tbsp	Natural Yogurt

Preparation

1. Heat the **oats** with the **milk**, grated **apple** and 50ml water. Bring to the boil.

2. Turn down the heat and simmer for 10 mins, or until the oats are cooked.

3. Serve scattered with **pecans**, **blueberries** and a tablespoon of **yogurt**.

285 Cals

1 5-a-day

3g Fibre

5g SatFat

15g Fat

9g Protein

31g Carbs

Weight | 215g

Smoked Salmon & Egg

A sub-300-calorie take on eggs royale. Can't go wrong with the tried and tested egg & salmon combo!

Ingredients

1	**Egg**
1 slice	**Rye Bread**
⅛	**Cucumber** (sliced)
1	handful **Rocket**
50g	**Smoked Salmon** (sliced)
¼	**Lemon** (juice only)
1 sprig	**Dill** (chopped)

Preparation

1. Poach the **egg** in boiling water (with or without vinegar) for 4 mins.
2. Toast the **rye bread**, then layer with **cucumber**, **rocket**, **salmon** and egg.
3. Serve drizzled with **lemon juice** and sprinkled with **dill**.

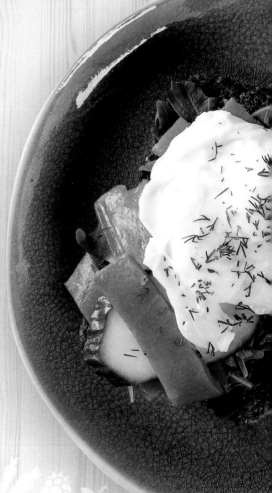

24g Carbs	26g Protein	11g Fat	3g SatFat	4g Fibre

Weight | 215g

1 5-a-day	290 Cals

Mushroom Pepper Omelette

Short on time? Whip up a mouth-watering cheesy omelette in minutes!

Ingredients

40g	**Mushrooms** (thinly sliced)
¼	**Red Pepper** (thinly sliced)
1 tsp	**Olive Oil**
1	handful **Spinach**
2	**Eggs** (whisked)
8	**Cherry Tomatoes** (on the vine)
10g	**Cheddar Cheese** (grated)
1 sprig	**Parsley** (chopped)

Preparation

1. Pan fry the **mushrooms** and **pepper** in 1 tsp **oil**, until soft.

2. Add the **spinach** and cook for a further minute.

3. Pour the **eggs** over the vegetables in the pan.

4. When the egg mixture starts to firm up, drop in the **cherry tomatoes** to cook at the side of the pan.

5. Sprinkle the **cheese** and **parsley** on top. Cook for a further 2 mins, then serve.

295 Cals

2 5-a-day

2g Fibre

6g SatFat

19g Fat

20g Protein

6g Carbs

Weight | 300g

Egg White & Baked Beans

This satisfying slice is our highest-fibre breakfast, with 11g fibre and 3 of your 5-a-day

Ingredients

80g	**Cannellini Beans** (tinned)
40g	**Kidney Beans** (tinned)
120g	**Chopped Tomatoes** (tinned)
1/3	**Red Onion** (diced)
2 tsp	**Demerara Sugar**
1 tbsp	**White Wine Vinegar**
2	**Egg Whites**
1 slice	**Sourdough Bread** (small)
1 sprig	**Parsley** (chopped)

Preparation

1. Gently cook the **beans**, **tomatoes**, **onion**, **sugar** and **vinegar** in a pan, with 50ml water, for 25 mins.

2. Meanwhile, scramble the **egg whites** on a high heat (with no oil) until white and moist.

3. Serve on the **bread** and top with **parsley**.

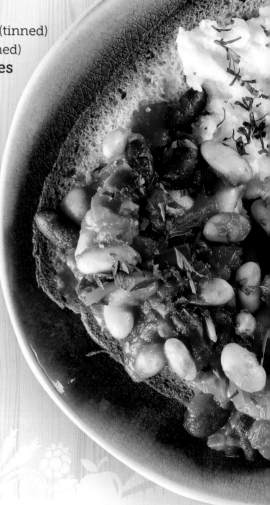

51g	22g	2g	0g	11g
Carbs	Protein	Fat	SatFat	Fibre

Weight | 310g

3	310
5-a-day	Cals

Wild Rice Kedgeree

This delicious spicy mishmash is our highest-protein
breakfast, thanks to the haddock and egg

Ingredients

35g	uncooked **Wild Rice** (rinsed)
70g	**Haddock** (raw fillet, sustainable)
150ml	**Milk** (whole)
1/8	**Onion** (diced)
1 tsp	**Olive Oil**
1 tsp	**Curry Paste**
1 sprig	**Coriander** (large, chopped)
1	**Egg** (hard boiled, quartered)
1/4	**Lemon** (juice only)

Preparation

1. Cook the **rice** according
   to pack instructions.

2. In another pan, poach the
   haddock in **milk** for 4 mins, or
   until the flesh turns opaque.

3. Meanwhile, pan fry the **onion** in
   1 tsp **oil** with the **curry paste** for a
   couple of minutes. Then add half
   the **coriander** and cook gently
   for a further few minutes.

4. Drain the rice and combine
   with the onion mixture.

5. Flake the haddock into the rice, then top
   with the **egg** and remaining coriander.

6. Finish with a squeeze of **lemon juice**.

315 Cals

1/2 5-a-day

2g Fibre

2g SatFat

11g Fat

26g Protein

29g Carbs

Weight | 270g

Okra & Lentil Curry

Oh my goodness... this nutritious curry has 4 of your 5-a-day for only 255 calories!

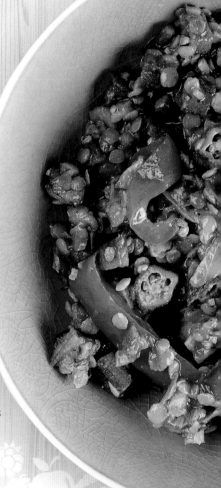

Ingredients

80g	**Aubergine** (cubed)	
½	**Red Pepper** (sliced)	
1 tsp	**Olive Oil**	
¼	**Onion** (sliced)	
¼ tsp	**Black Mustard Seeds**	
1 clove	**Garlic** (minced)	
1 tsp	**Curry Paste**	
80g	**Okra** (chopped)	
40g	dried **Red Split Lentils**	
200ml	**Vegetable Stock** (½ cube)	
1 sprig	**Coriander** (large, chopped)	

Preparation

1. Mix the **aubergine** and **pepper** with 1 tsp **oil** and bake at 180°C for 25 mins.
2. Meanwhile, dry fry the **onion** until soft, then add the **mustard seeds**, **garlic**, **curry paste** and **okra**.
3. Stir in the **lentils** and **stock**. Bring to the boil, then simmer for 20 mins or until the lentils are cooked.
4. Fold in the roasted veggies, top with **coriander**, and serve.

35g Carbs	14g Protein	7g Fat	1g SatFat	12g Fibre

Weight | 350g

4 5-a-day	255 Cals

Thai Green Prawn Curry

Anyone curbing their carbs will go crazy
for this creamy coconut curry

Ingredients

1 tbsp	Thai Green Curry Paste
1 tsp	Olive Oil
1/3	Courgette (sliced lengthways)
40g	Green Beans (quartered)
1 tbsp	Coconut Cream
1 tsp	Fish Sauce
100g	King Prawns (raw)
40g	Peas
1 sprig	Coriander (large, chopped)

Preparation

1. Heat the **curry paste** in 1 tsp **oil** for 1 min, before adding 50ml water to make a thin paste.
2. Add the **courgette** and **green beans**, cook for a minute, then stir in the **coconut cream** and **fish sauce**.
3. Bring to the boil, then combine the **prawns** and **peas** with the mixture.
4. Turn down the heat and simmer until the prawns are cooked.
5. Serve scattered with the **coriander**.

280 Cals   **2** 5-a-day

4g Fibre   **10g** SatFat   **16g** Fat   **24g** Protein   **9g** Carbs

Weight | 250g

Jamaican Chicken Curry

The ultimate curry... with a whopping 36g protein, 4 of your 5-a-day, and nearly half your daily fibre needs!

Ingredients

1 tsp	**Curry Powder**
1 tsp	**Olive Oil**
100g	**Chicken Breast** (raw, skinless, cubed)
⅓	**Red Onion** (thinly sliced)
½	**Red Chilli** (chopped)
120g	**Tomato** (chopped)
¼	**Red Pepper** (sliced)
¼	**Yellow Pepper** (sliced)
80g	**Natural Yogurt**
100ml	**Chicken Stock** (½ cube)
80g	**Kidney Beans** (tinned)
¼	**Mango** (cubed)
1 sprig	**Coriander** (large, chopped)

Preparation

1. Coat the chicken in **curry powder**. Heat 1 tsp **oil** in a pan, add the **chicken** and brown for 3 mins.

2. Stir in the **onion**, **chilli**, **tomato** and **peppers**. Fry for a further 5 mins.

3. Pour in the **yogurt** and **stock**. Bring to the boil, then simmer until the chicken is cooked.

4. Add the **beans** and **mango**. Cook gently until the beans are warmed through.

5. Sprinkle with chopped **coriander** to serve.

35g Carbs	36g Protein	10g Fat	3g SatFat	14g Fibre

Weight | 500g

4 5-a-day   **360** Cals

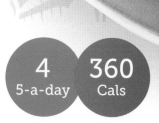

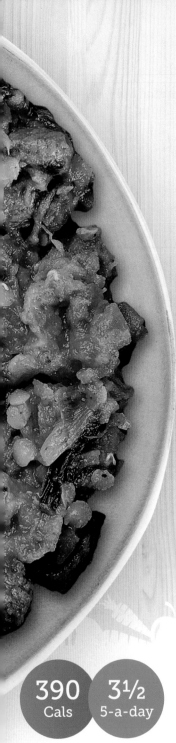

Lamb Dhansak

Like lamb? You'll love this hearty bowlful!

Ingredients

70g	**Stewing Lamb** (raw, diced)
1 pod	**Cardamom** (seeds only, ground)
pinch	**Coriander** (ground)
pinch	**Cumin** (ground)
pinch	**Turmeric** (ground)
¼	**Onion** (diced)
1 inch	**Ginger** (grated)
1 clove	**Garlic** (minced)
½	**Red Chilli** (sliced)
150g	**Chopped Tomatoes** (tinned)
80g	**Butternut Squash** (cubed)
40g	dried **Red Split Lentils**
200ml	**Beef Stock** (½ cube)
2	handfuls **Spinach**
1 sprig	**Coriander** (large, chopped)

Preparation

1. Coat the **lamb** in the **dry spices** and dry fry until browned and aromatic.

2. Add the **onion** and fry for 5 mins until soft.

3. Stir in the **ginger**, **garlic** and sliced **chilli** and cook for a further 2 mins.

4. Mix through the **tomatoes**, **squash**, **lentils** and **stock**, and bring to the boil.

5. Simmer the mixture for 25 mins, or until the lentils are cooked and the curry is thick.

6. Fold in the **spinach** and allow to wilt. Serve topped with the fresh **coriander**.

390 Cals

3½ 5-a-day

8g Fibre

5g SatFat

12g Fat

33g Protein

41g Carbs

Weight | 410g

Sweet Potato Curry

A full-flavoured veggie delight to tickle your taste buds in all the right places!

Ingredients

⅓	**Red Onion** (thinly sliced)
1 tsp	**Olive Oil**
1 tbsp	**Coconut Cream**
1 tbsp	**Curry Paste**
80g	**Cauliflower** (small florets)
1	**Red Chilli** (sliced)
1 inch	**Ginger** (grated)
80g	**Sweet Potato** (cubed)
80g	**Chickpeas** (tinned)
150ml	**Vegetable Stock** (½ cube)
80g	**Tomato** (chopped)
1 sprig	**Coriander** (large, chopped)

Preparation

1. Fry the **onion** in 1 tsp **oil** until soft. Stir in the **coconut cream** and **curry paste**.
2. Add the **cauliflower**, **chilli**, **ginger**, **sweet potato** and **chickpeas**. Cook for 5 mins.
3. Pour in the **stock**, along with the **tomato** and half of the **coriander**.
4. Bring to the boil, then simmer for 20 mins, or until the potato is cooked.
5. Serve sprinkled with the remaining coriander.

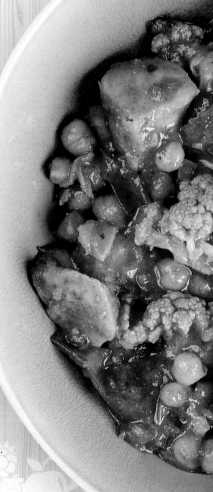

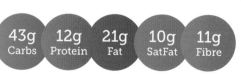

43g Carbs **12g** Protein **21g** Fat **10g** SatFat **11g** Fibre

3½ 5-a-day **395** Cals

Weight | 620g

Cauliflower Risotto

Slurp up this soupy, riceless risotto -
around half the calories of normal risotto!

Ingredients

¼	**Onion** (sliced)	
1 tsp	**Olive Oil**	
80g	**Mushrooms** (sliced)	
1 clove	**Garlic** (minced)	
160g	**Cauliflower** (grated)	
150ml	**Vegetable Stock** (½ cube)	
40g	**Petit Pois**	
1 sprig	**Thyme** (leaves, chopped)	
1 sprig	**Rosemary** (leaves, chopped)	
40g	**Greek Yogurt**	
20g	**Parmesan** (grated)	

Preparation

1. Fry the **onion** in 1 tsp **oil** for 1 min on a medium heat. Add the **mushrooms** and cook for 4 mins.

2. Next, stir in the **garlic** and **cauliflower**. Fry for 2 mins, then add the **stock** and **peas**.

3. Bring to the boil and simmer for 5 mins.

4. Sprinkle in the **thyme** and **rosemary**, and cook for 1 min, stirring in the **yogurt** and **parmesan**.

5. Remove from the heat and serve.

265 Cals

3 5-a-day

7g Fibre

7g SatFat

15g Fat

17g Protein

17g Carbs

Weight | 330g

Quinoa Stuffed Mushrooms

The quinoa in this dish is a great source of plant-based protein

Ingredients

1/3	**Red Onion** (finely chopped)
1 tsp	**Olive Oil**
50g	**Ricotta**
80g	cooked **Quinoa**
1 sprig	**Parsley** (large, chopped)
1/2 tsp	**Oregano** (dried)
2	**Portobello Mushrooms**
8	**Cherry Tomatoes** (on the vine)
1	large handful **Watercress**

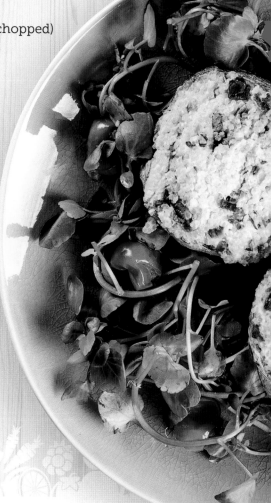

Preparation

1. Fry the **onion** in 1 tsp **oil** until soft.

2. Mix the onion with the **ricotta**, cooked **quinoa**, **herbs**, salt and pepper.

3. Stuff the **mushrooms** with the ricotta mixture and roast, along with the **tomatoes** (on the vine), for 20 mins at 200°C.

4. Serve on a bed of **watercress**.

24g Carbs	13g Protein	13g Fat	4g SatFat	7g Fibre

Weight | 330g

2½ 5-a-day

265 Cals

Pollock & Chickpeas

Pollock packs a protein punch in this winning combination

Ingredients

140g	**Pollock** (raw fillet)
¼	**Lemon** (juice only)
8	**Cherry Tomatoes**
1 tsp	**Olive Oil**
80g	**Chickpeas** (tinned)
pinch	**Sumac** (large)
4	handfuls **Spinach**

Preparation

1. Season **fish** with **lemon juice** and salt & pepper. Place on a baking tray, surrounded by **tomatoes**.

2. Bake for 12 mins at 200°C, or until the fish is cooked.

3. Meanwhile, heat 1 tsp **oil** in a pan and add the **chickpeas** and **sumac**, frying for 3 mins.

4. Add the **spinach** and cook for a further 2 mins.

5. Serve the fish on top of the chickpeas, spinach and tomatoes, drizzling any pan juices over the top.

270 Cals

4 5-a-day

8g Fibre

1g SatFat

9g Fat

32g Protein

17g Carbs

Weight | 305g

Huevos Rancheros

A delicious Mexican dish to help you eat a rainbow of nutrients

Ingredients

1/3	**Red Onion** (finely chopped)
1/2	**Carrot** (finely chopped)
1/4	**Red Pepper** (diced)
1/4	**Yellow Pepper** (diced)
pinch	**Cumin** (ground)
pinch	**Smoked Paprika**
1 tsp	**Olive Oil**
100g	**Chopped Tomatoes** (tinned)
1 clove	**Garlic** (minced)
1	handful **Kale** (chopped)
2	**Eggs**
1 sprig	**Coriander** (large, chopped)

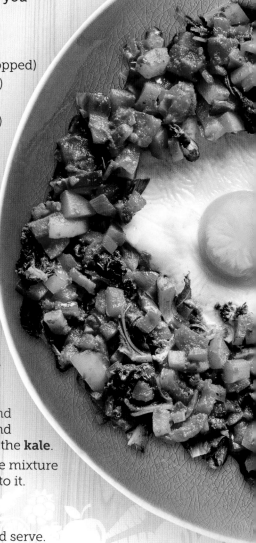

Preparation

1. Fry the **onion**, **carrot**, **peppers**, **cumin** and **paprika** in 1 tsp **oil** for 5 mins, until softened.

2. Pour in the **tomatoes**, **garlic** and 50ml water. Bring to the boil and simmer for 5 mins, then stir in the **kale**.

3. Make a well in the middle of the mixture and carefully crack the **eggs** into it.

4. Put the pan in the oven at 200°C for 5 mins.

5. Sprinkle with the **coriander** and serve.

15g Carbs	19g Protein	16g Fat	4g SatFat	6g Fibre

Weight | 250g

3 5-a-day

275 Cals

Cheesy Cod Fillets

Crunchy, cheesy, fishy, yummy!

Ingredients

140g	**Cod** (raw fillet, sustainable)
40g	**Leek** (thinly sliced)
40g	**Fennel** (thinly sliced)
1 tsp	**Olive Oil**
½ slice	**Wholemeal Bread** (breadcrumbs)
25g	**Cheddar Cheese** (grated)
1 sprig	**Parsley** (large, chopped)
80g	**Kale** (blanched)

Preparation

1. Grill the **cod** for 5 mins.
2. Meanwhile, fry the **leek** and **fennel** in 1 tsp **oil** until softened.
3. Combine the **breadcrumbs** with the **cheese** and **parsley**.
4. Spoon the veg onto the cod, season, then cover with the cheese mixture.
5. Grill for a further 3 mins until golden, and serve on a bed of **kale**.

325 Cals

2 5-a-day

7g Fibre

7g SatFat

16g Fat

36g Protein

10g Carbs

Weight | 275g

Moroccan Veg & Chickpeas

A spicy concoction, delivering a massive 7½ portions of veg and over half your daily fibre requirements. Tuck in!

Ingredients

80g	**Aubergine**	(cubed)
½	**Beetroot**	(raw, cubed)
½	**Carrot**	(chopped)
80g	**Cauliflower**	(florets, halved)
⅓	**Courgette**	(cubed)
⅓	**Red Onion**	(wedges)
¼	**Red Pepper**	(chopped)
¼	**Yellow Pepper**	(chopped)
2 cloves	**Garlic**	(skin on)
2 tsp	**Olive Oil**	
pinch	**Chilli Flakes, Coriander Seeds, Cumin Seeds, Nigella Seeds & Sumac**	
4	**Cherry Tomatoes**	
100g	**Chickpeas**	(tinned)
1	handful **Kale**	
5	**Mint** leaves	(torn)
1 sprig	**Coriander**	(large, chopped)

Preparation

1. Mix the **veg** (except the kale and tomatoes) with 1 tsp **oil**, **garlic** and **spices**. Bake at 200°C for 20 mins.
2. When cooked, squeeze the roasted garlic out of its skin and fry with the **tomatoes** in 1 tsp oil for 1 min.
3. Add 100ml water, bring to the boil, simmer until reduced.
4. Stir in the **chickpeas**, adding the **kale** after 1 min.
5. Plate up the roasted veg surrounded by the chickpea mixture, and scatter with **mint** and **coriander** to serve.

39g Carbs	15g Protein	13g Fat	2g SatFat	18g Fibre		7½ 5-a-day	325 Cals

Weight | 415g

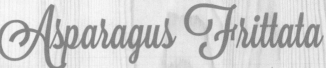

Asparagus Frittata

This low-carb lunch can be eaten hot or cold,
making it perfect for taking to work

Ingredients

¼	**Onion** (sliced)
1 tsp	**Olive Oil**
80g	**Asparagus Tips** (chopped)
20g	**Sun-dried Tomatoes** (chopped)
1 sprig	**Parsley** (large, chopped)
3	**Eggs** (whisked)

Preparation

1. Using a small oven-proof frying pan, gently fry the **onion** for 3 mins in 1 tsp **oil**.

2. Add the **asparagus**, **tomatoes** and **parsley**, and cook for 2 mins to soften.

3. Turn the heat up until the pan sizzles, then add the **eggs** and cook for 2 mins.

4. Place the pan in the oven at 200°C for a further 8 mins, until the frittata is set, then serve.

340 Cals

1½ 5-a-day

4g Fibre

5g SatFat

23g Fat

26g Protein

6g Carbs

Weight | 240g

Fish Pie

A comforting dinner for those evenings when your taste buds need a bit of TLC!

Ingredients

120g	**Cauliflower** (small florets)
120g	**Butternut Squash** (cubed)
10g	**Parmesan** (grated)
¼	**Onion** (diced)
½	**Carrot** (finely chopped)
1 tsp	**Olive Oil**
1	handful **Spinach**
40g	**Tomato** (chopped)
1 sprig	**Dill** (chopped)
1 sprig	**Parsley** (large, chopped)
2 tsp	**Whipping Cream**
70g	**Pollock** (raw fillet, cubed)
70g	**Prawns** (raw)
¼	**Lemon** (juice only)

Preparation

1. Steam the **cauliflower** and **squash** until tender. Mash with **parmesan**, salt & pepper.
2. Fry the **onion** and **carrot** in 1 tsp **oil** until soft. Stir in the **spinach** and allow to wilt.
3. Add the **tomato**, a splash of water and the **herbs**.
4. Cook until the tomato starts to break down, then fold in the **cream**.
5. Place the **fish** and **prawns** in a baking dish. Spoon the vegetable mixture evenly over the top.
6. Drizzle with **lemon juice** and top with the cauliflower mash. Bake at 180°C for 20 mins and serve.

24g Carbs	33g Protein	13g Fat	5g SatFat	8g Fibre

Weight | 400g

4½ 5-a-day

340 Cals

Dijon Chicken with Mash

If you think mashed potato is marvellous, wait until you taste this parsnip & bean mash-up!

Ingredients

1	**Parsnip** (chunks)
40g	**Cannellini Beans**
100g	**Chicken Breast** (raw, skinless, diced)
1 tsp	**Olive Oil**
200ml	**Chicken Stock** (½ cube)
1 tsp	**Dijon Mustard**
25g	**Cream Cheese**
80g	**Broccoli** (florets)
80g	**Asparagus** (halved)
2 sprigs	**Tarragon** (chopped)

Preparation

1. Boil **parsnip** (using water from cold). Simmer for 12 mins until soft, adding the **beans** for the final minute. Drain and mash.

2. Fry the **chicken** on a high heat in 1 tsp **oil** for 5 mins, or until golden. Transfer to a warm plate.

3. In the same pan, boil the **stock**, whisking in the **mustard** and **cheese**. Return chicken to the pan and simmer for 10 mins.

4. Meanwhile, boil or steam the **broccoli** and **asparagus** for 3 mins, until tender.

5. Serve sprinkled with **tarragon** and drizzled with sauce.

355 Cals

3½ 5-a-day

11g Fibre

5g SatFat

14g Fat

36g Protein

22g Carbs

Weight | 365g

Turkey Meatballs

An interesting, low-calorie alternative
to a traditional roast dinner

Ingredients

1/8	**Onion**
1 clove	**Garlic**
6	**Basil** leaves
1 sprig	**Thyme** (leaves)
1	**Egg**
1	handful **Rocket**
100g	**Turkey Mince** (raw)
80g	**Sweet Potato** (cubed)
1 tsp	**Olive Oil**
1 sprig	**Rosemary** (leaves, chopped)
8	**Cherry Tomatoes**
120g	**Green Beans**

Preparation

1. Whizz the **onion**, **garlic**, **basil**, **thyme**, **egg** and **rocket** in a food processor and transfer to a bowl.
2. Use your hands to combine the **mince** with the herb mixture and form into small balls.
3. On a baking tray, coat the **sweet potato** with 1 tsp **oil** and sprinkle with **rosemary**.
4. Place the meatballs on the same tray and cook at 200°C for 20 mins.
5. Add the **tomatoes** to the tray and roast for a further 8 mins.
6. Meanwhile, boil or steam the **beans** for 3 mins. Assemble on a plate and enjoy!

26g Carbs
36g Protein
12g Fat
3g SatFat
9g Fibre

2½ 5-a-day
355 Cals

Weight | 280g

Chickpea Patties

Keep your energy flowing smoothly with the slow release carbs in these pleasant patties

Ingredients

80g	**Chickpeas** (tinned)
1 clove	**Garlic**
1/3	**Courgette**
1 sprig	**Coriander**
pinch	**Cumin** (ground)
1	**Egg**
2 tbsp	**Oats**
1 tsp	**Olive Oil**
8	**Cherry Tomatoes**
1	handful **Spinach**
1/4	**Avocado** (sliced)

Preparation

1. Blitz the **chickpeas**, **garlic**, **courgette**, **coriander**, **cumin**, **egg** and **oats** in a food processor.

2. Use the mixture to form patties, then chill for 1 hour, until firm.

3. Fry the patties in 1 tsp **oil** on a low heat, until crisp on both sides. Set aside on a warm plate.

4. In the same pan, cook the **tomatoes** until they start to burst.

5. To serve, layer the **spinach** and patties, topped with sliced **avocado** and tomatoes.

355 Cals

3½ 5-a-day

10g Fibre

4g SatFat

20g Fat

18g Protein

26g Carbs

Weight | 340g

Tuna & Roasted Veg

Get all 5 of your 5-a-day (and 41g protein!) with this succulent tuna steak on a colourful bed of veg

Ingredients

80g	**Aubergine** (cubed)
160g	**Butternut Squash** (cubed)
1/3	**Courgette** (cubed)
2 cloves	**Garlic** (in skin)
pinch	**Oregano** (dried)
1/2	**Red Pepper** (cubed)
1 sprig	**Rosemary** (leaves, chopped)
1/2	**Yellow Pepper** (cubed)
2 tsp	**Olive Oil**
140g	**Tuna Steak** (fresh)
1 tsp	**Cajun Seasoning**
1/2	**Lime** (juice only)

Preparation

1. Combine **all the ingredients** (except the tuna, lime juice, Cajun seasoning and half the oil) and roast at 200°C for 20 mins.
2. Meanwhile, season the **tuna** on each side with the **Cajun seasoning**.
3. Fry the tuna in the remaining 1 tsp **oil** for 2 mins on each side.
4. Drizzle the **lime juice** over the tuna towards the end of cooking.
5. When the vegetables are cooked, squeeze the garlic out of its skin.
6. Serve the tuna on the veg, drizzled with pan juices.

26g Carbs	41g Protein	10g Fat	2g SatFat	11g Fibre

5 5-a-day

355 Cals

Weight | 445g

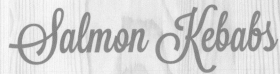

Salmon Kebabs

These low-cal kebabs are perfect for the BBQ

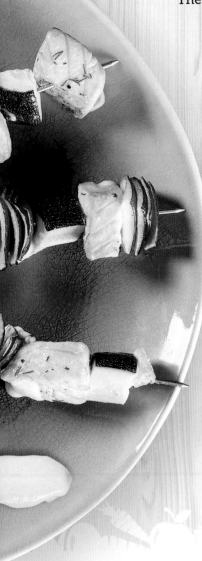

Ingredients

1 tsp	Olive Oil
1/2 tsp	Dijon Mustard
1	Lemon (juice only)
140g	Salmon (raw fillet, cubed)
1/3	Courgette (cubed)
1/3	Red Onion (cubed)
1/2	Yellow Pepper (cubed)
40g	Natural Yogurt
1 sprig	Dill (finely chopped)

Preparation

1. Mix 1 tsp **oil**, **mustard**, salt & pepper and half the **lemon juice** in a bowl.

2. Coat the **salmon** with the mixture and allow to marinate in the fridge for 30 mins.

3. Dry fry the **courgette**, **onion** and **pepper** for 4 mins until charred. Thread onto skewers with the salmon, to make kebabs.

4. Bake on a tray at 200°C for 8 mins, or until the salmon is cooked.

5. Meanwhile, mix the **yogurt**, remaining lemon juice, and **dill** in a bowl.

6. Serve the kebabs drizzled with the yogurt dressing.

375 Cals

3 5-a-day

4g Fibre

5g SatFat

21g Fat

36g Protein

12g Carbs

Weight | 300g

Chicken, Kale & Chorizo

Stuff yourself with this heavenly dish (and an impressive 47g protein)

Ingredients

40g	**Roasted Red Pepper** (from jar, chopped)
25g	**Cream Cheese**
6	**Basil** leaves (torn)
150g	**Chicken Breast** (raw, skinless)
½ tsp	**Olive Oil**
25g	**Chorizo** (small cubes)
4	handfuls **Kale** (chopped)

Preparation

1. Mix the **pepper** with the **cheese** and **basil**. Cut a pocket into the **chicken breast** and spoon in the cheese mixture.

2. Rub ½ tsp **oil** over the chicken and bake for 18 mins at 200°C, or until the chicken is thoroughly cooked.

3. Gently dry fry the **chorizo** until oils are released. Turn the heat up, add a good splash of water and the **kale**.

4. Cook until the kale has wilted, then serve topped with the chicken.

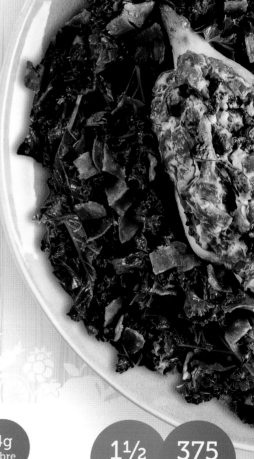

5g Carbs	47g Protein	19g Fat	8g SatFat	4g Fibre

Weight | 275g

1½ 5-a-day	375 Cals

Mexican Chicken Mole

Chilli and chocolate in the mole sauce
spice up this flavoursome fiesta!

Ingredients

2/3	**Red Onion** (sliced)
1/2	**Red Pepper** (sliced)
1 tsp	**Olive Oil**
2 cloves	**Garlic** (minced)
200g	**Chopped Tomatoes** (tinned)
80g	**Mixed Beans**
1 tbsp	**Mole Sauce**
150g	**Chicken Thighs** (raw, skinless, boneless)
1 sprig	**Parsley** (large, chopped)

Preparation

1. Gently fry the **onion** and **pepper** in 1 tsp **oil** for 10 mins, until soft.

2. Add the **garlic** and cook for a further minute.

3. Stir in the **tomatoes**, **beans**, **mole sauce** and 150ml water, and bring to the boil.

4. Add the **chicken** and simmer for at least 30 mins, ensuring the chicken is thoroughly cooked.

5. Serve sprinkled with the chopped **parsley**.

390 Cals	4 5-a-day	12g Fibre	2g SatFat	10g Fat	41g Protein	31g Carbs

Weight | 400g

Triple Tomato Salad

If you like tomatoes, why not have them three ways?

Ingredients

160g	**Tomato** (sliced)
¼	**Lime** (juice only)
8	**Cherry Tomatoes** (halved)
30g	**Sun-dried Tomatoes** (chopped)

Dressing

6	**Basil** leaves (torn)
2 sprigs	**Parsley** (chopped)
1 sprig	**Tarragon** (chopped)

Preparation

1. Arrange the **sliced tomato** on a plate and squeeze over the **lime juice**.

2. Mix the **cherry tomatoes** and **sun-dried tomatoes** and place on top of the sliced tomato.

3. Serve with chopped **herbs** and salt & pepper.

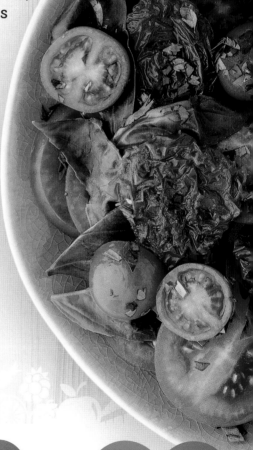

11g Carbs	3g Protein	4g Fat	1g SatFat	5g Fibre

Weight | 285g

2½ 5-a-day

95 Cals

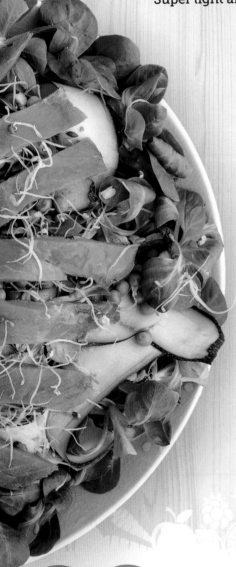

Sprouty Salmon Salad

Super light and refreshing with only 140 calories

Ingredients

20g	**Alfalfa Sprouts**
1/3	**Courgette** (ribboned)
1 clove	**Garlic** (minced)
2	handfuls **Lambs Lettuce**
1/4	**Lemon** (juice only)
40g	**Petit Pois** (cooked)
50g	**Smoked Salmon** (strips)

Preparation

1. Combine **all the ingredients** except the salmon.

2. Lay the **salmon** on top of the salad and season with pepper.

140 Cals

2 5-a-day

3g Fibre

1g SatFat

5g Fat

17g Protein

6g Carbs

Weight | 230g

Olive Steak Salad

A perfect combination of steak, olives and sprouts

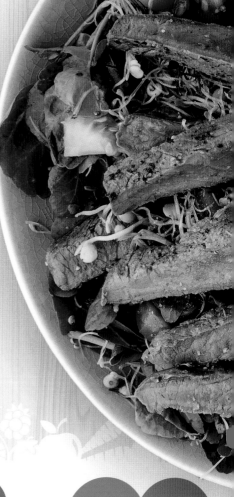

Ingredients

1 tsp	**Olive Oil**
100g	**Beef Sirloin** (raw, lean)
40g	**Alfalfa Sprouts**
1 sprig	**Dill** (finely chopped)
8	**Olives** (small, chopped)
80g	**Tomato** (chopped)
1	large handful **Watercress**
¼	**Lemon** (juice only)

Preparation

1. Heat the **oil** in a pan over a medium-high heat and fry the **steak** for 2 mins each side. Remove the pan from the heat.

2. Mix **all the salad ingredients** (except the lemon juice) and place on a plate.

3. Slice the steak into strips, and lay on top of the salad.

4. Drizzle with juices from the pan and the **lemon juice**.

3g Carbs	26g Protein	12g Fat	3g SatFat	3g Fibre

Weight | 285g

2 5-a-day

225 Cals

Prawn & Avocado Salad

Sweet pineapple and salty olives make for a great combination

Ingredients

¼	**Avocado** (cubed)
8	**Cherry Tomatoes** (quartered)
1 sprig	**Dill** (finely chopped)
100g	**King Prawns** (cooked)
8	**Olives** (small, halved)
2 sprigs	**Parsley** (finely chopped)
40g	**Pineapple** (chopped)
1	**Spring Onion** (sliced)
40g	**Little Gem Lettuce**

Dressing

¼	**Lemon** (juice only)
1 tsp	**Olive Oil** (extra virgin)

Preparation

1. Mix **all the salad ingredients** together, except the lettuce.
2. Whisk the **dressing** until well combined and stir through the salad.
3. Lay a bed of **lettuce** on a plate and top with the salad mixture.

230 Cals

3 5-a-day

4g Fibre

3g SatFat

14g Fat

18g Protein

6g Carbs

Weight | 355g

Tuna & Bean Salad

Packed with 26g protein for only 265 calories

Ingredients

40g	**Asparagus Tips** (blanched)
80g	**Cannellini Beans** (tinned)
1/3	**Red Onion** (thinly sliced)
2	handfuls **Spinach**
70g	**Tuna** (tinned)

Dressing

1 sprig	**Dill** (chopped)
1/2 clove	**Garlic** (crushed)
2 tsp	**Olive Oil** (extra virgin)
1 sprig	**Parsley** (large)
1 tbsp	**White Wine Vinegar**

Preparation

1. Mix **all the salad ingredients** and season with salt & pepper.
2. Whisk the **dressing** until well combined and gently stir through the salad.

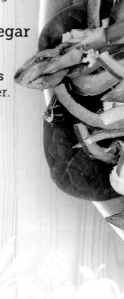

17g Carbs	26g Protein	10g Fat	2g SatFat	8g Fibre

Weight | 300g

2½ 5-a-day

265 Cals

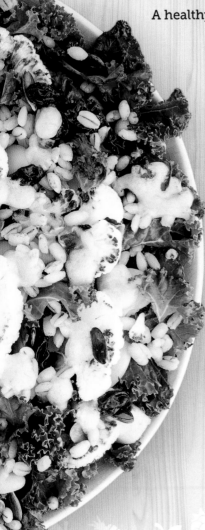

Warm Cauli Salad

A healthy, hearty dish with raisin flavourbombs

Ingredients

1 tsp	**Olive Oil**
80g	**Cauliflower** florets (sliced)
2	handfuls **Kale**
80g	**Butter Beans** (tinned)
2 sprigs	**Parsley** (chopped)
80g	cooked **Pearl Barley**
1 tbsp	**Pumpkin Seeds**
1 tbsp	**Raisins** (heaped)

Dressing

½ tsp	**Dijon Mustard**
¼	**Lemon** (juice only)
1 tsp	**Olive Oil** (extra virgin)

Preparation

1. Whisk the **dressing** until well combined.
2. Heat 1 tsp **oil** in a pan and add the **cauliflower**. After 3 mins, add the **kale** and cook for a further 2 mins.
3. Add the **remaining ingredients** to the warm vegetables and serve drizzled with dressing.

275 Cals

3 5-a-day

9g Fibre

2g SatFat

14g Fat

11g Protein

27g Carbs

Weight | 255g

Crab & Asparagus Salad

A light, refreshing and summery salad

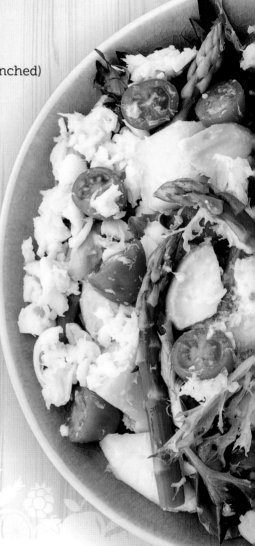

Ingredients

80g	**Asparagus Tips** (blanched)
¼	**Avocado** (cubed)
8	**Cherry Tomatoes** (halved)
100g	**Crab** (tinned)
¼	**Mango** (cubed)
1	handful **Mixed Salad Leaves**

Dressing

¼	**Lemon** (juice only)
½	**Lemon** (peel only, grated)
2 tsp	**Olive Oil** (extra virgin)
2 sprigs	**Parsley** (chopped)

Preparation

1. Combine **all the salad ingredients**.
2. Stir together the **dressing** and toss through the salad.

12g Carbs	23g Protein	16g Fat	3g SatFat	7g Fibre

Weight | 385g

3½ 5-a-day

280 Cals

Mustard Chicken Salad

With 33g protein in one dish, this chicken and wholegrain mustard fusion is a great way to fill up

Ingredients

80g	**Black Eye Beans** (tinned)
4	**Cherry Tomatoes** (quartered)
80g	**Chicken Breast** (grilled, sliced)
2	handfuls **Mixed Salad Leaves**
1 sprig	**Tarragon** (chopped)

Dressing

2 tsp	**Olive Oil** (extra virgin)
1 tsp	**White Wine Vinegar**
1 tsp	**Wholegrain Mustard**

Preparation

1. Whisk the **dressing** together until mixed well.
2. Combine the **salad ingredients** and gently stir through the dressing.
3. Season with salt & pepper and serve.

305 Cals

2 5-a-day

5g Fibre

2g SatFat

11g Fat

33g Protein

16g Carbs

Weight | 260g

Warm Squash Salad

Smoky houmous is a great addition to this kale and squash salad

Ingredients

80g	**Butternut Squash** (cubed)
½	**Yellow Pepper** (sliced)
1 tsp	**Olive Oil**
2	handfuls **Kale**
1 tbsp	**Pumpkin Seeds**

Dressing

80g	**Chickpeas** (tinned)
½ tsp	**Cumin** (ground)
1 clove	**Garlic** (minced)
¼	**Lemon** (juice only)
½ tsp	**Smoked Paprika**
2 tsp	**Tahini**
2 tbsp	**Water**

Preparation

1. Bake the **squash** and **pepper** at 180°C with 1 tsp **oil** for 20 mins.
2. Add the **kale** and cook for 5 mins more.
3. Meanwhile, blitz the **dressing** in a blender to make the houmous.
4. Serve the salad topped with the houmous & **pumpkin seeds**.

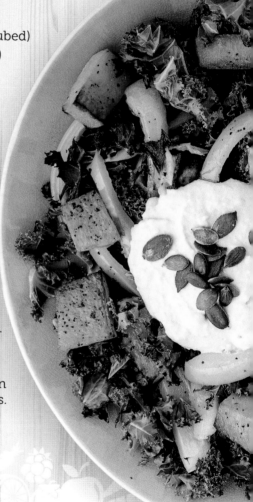

28g	14g	18g	3g	12g
Carbs	Protein	Fat	SatFat	Fibre

Weight | 315g

3½	320
5-a-day	Cals

Bean & Cheese Salad

A large plate of yumminess with all your
5-a-day and only 12g carbs!

Ingredients

8	**Cherry Tomatoes** (halved)
¼	**Cucumber** (cubed)
25g	**Goat's Cheese** (cubed)
80g	**Green Beans** (blanched, halved)
8	**Olives** (small, chopped)
40g	**Radishes** (sliced)
80g	**Soya Beans** (cooked)

Dressing

1 tbsp	**Capers**
¼	**Lemon** (juice only)
2 tsp	**Olive Oil** (extra virgin)
2 sprigs	**Rosemary** (chopped)

Preparation

1. Thoroughly mix **all the salad ingredients**.
2. Whisk the **dressing** and drizzle over the salad.

350 Cals

5 5-a-day

10g Fibre

7g SatFat

24g Fat

19g Protein

12g Carbs

Weight | 445g

Egg & Mackerel Salad

A creamy horseradish hit for the taste buds

Ingredients

2	handfuls	**Mixed Salad Leaves**
40g	**Asparagus Tips** (blanched)	
4	**Cherry Tomatoes** (halved)	
1	**Egg** (hard boiled, sliced)	
75g	**Smoked Mackerel**	

Dressing

1 tbsp	**Greek Yogurt**
1 clove	**Garlic** (minced)
¼	**Lemon** (juice only)
1 tsp	**Horseradish Sauce**

Preparation

1. Layer the **salad leaves** and **asparagus** on a plate, then top with the **tomatoes**, **egg** and **mackerel**.
2. Whisk the **dressing** until well combined and drizzle over the salad.
3. Season with salt & pepper and serve.

5g Carbs	28g Protein	26g Fat	6g SatFat	2g Fibre

Weight | 295g

1½ 5-a-day

370 Cals

Sticky Salmon Salad

At a whopping 37g, this is our highest protein salad
– so much goodness on one elegant plate!

Ingredients

150g	**Salmon** (raw fillet)
1	large handful **Watercress**
2	boiled **Beetroot** (sliced)
1/6	**Orange** (sliced)
1 tsp	**Sesame Seeds**

Dressing

1 clove	**Garlic** (minced)
1/2 inch	**Ginger** (minced)
1/4	**Lemon** (juice only)
1 tsp	**Sesame Oil**
1 tsp	**Soy Sauce**

Preparation

1. Place the **salmon** on a piece of foil, whisk the **dressing** and pour over the salmon. Fold the foil tightly to allow the fish to steam. Bake at 180°C for 15 mins, or until cooked.

2. On a plate, layer the **watercress**, **beetroot** and **orange** slices.

3. Place the sticky salmon fillet on top, pour over any juices from the foil and sprinkle with the **sesame seeds**.

385 Cals

2 5-a-day

3g Fibre

4g SatFat

21g Fat

37g Protein

13g Carbs

Weight | 310g

Thai Vegan Salad

No meat, no fish, no dairy... just 100% taste!

Ingredients

100g	**Tofu** (firm, cubed)
1 tsp	**Sesame Oil**
40g	**Beansprouts**
1	**Carrot** (matchsticks)
2 sprigs	**Coriander** (chopped)
1/3	**Courgette** (matchsticks)
1/4	**Cucumber** (matchsticks)
20g	**Radishes** (sliced)
40g	**Red Cabbage** (sliced)
2	**Spring Onions** (sliced)
1/4	**Yellow Pepper** (matchsticks)

Dressing

1 clove	**Garlic** (minced)
1/2 inch	**Ginger** (minced)
1/4	**Lime** (juice only)
2 tbsp	**Peanut Butter**
1 tbsp	**Rice Wine Vinegar**
1 tbsp	**Soy Sauce**

Preparation

1. Dry the **tofu** between paper towels. Rub with **oil** and bake for 45 mins at 180°C, until crispy.
2. Mix **all the other salad ingredients**.
3. Whisk the **dressing** and stir through the salad, topping with the tofu.

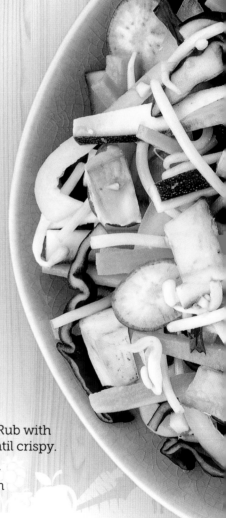

25g	20g	23g	4g	10g
Carbs	Protein	Fat	SatFat	Fibre

Weight | 560g

5	390
5-a-day	Cals

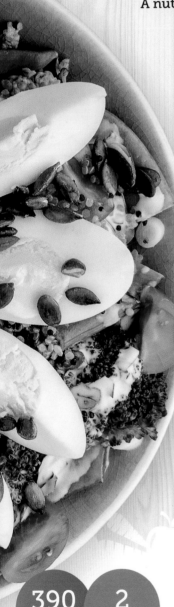

Egg & Quinoa Salad

A nutritious marriage of high-protein ingredients

Ingredients

40g	**Broccoli** (chopped)
4	**Cherry Tomatoes** (quartered)
80g	cooked **Quinoa**
1	**Spring Onion** (finely sliced)
40g	**Sugar Snap Peas** (halved)
1	**Egg** (hard boiled, quartered)
1 tbsp	**Pumpkin Seeds** (toasted)

Dressing

1 clove	**Garlic** (finely chopped)
¼	**Lemon** (juice only)
2 sprigs	**Parsley** (finely chopped)
1 tbsp	**Tahini**
1 tbsp	**Water**

Preparation

1. Boil or steam the **broccoli** for 3 mins, or until tender.

2. Mix **all the salad ingredients** except the egg and pumpkin seeds.

3. Whisk the **dressing** until well combined and stir through the salad.

4. Serve topped with the **egg** and scattered with **pumpkin seeds**.

390 Cals

2 5-a-day

9g Fibre

4g SatFat

22g Fat

24g Protein

25g Carbs

Weight | 370g

Roots & Lentil Salad

A curious combination of roasted roots
with a strawberry dressing

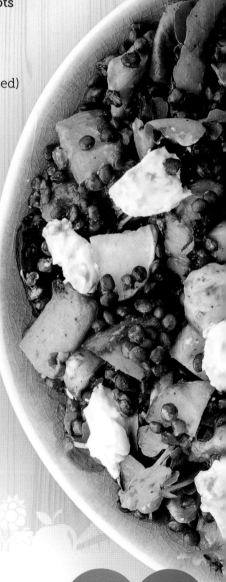

Ingredients

1	**Raw Beetroot** (peeled, cubed)
80g	**Butternut Squash** (peeled, cubed)
1	**Parsnip** (chopped)
1 clove	**Garlic** (minced)
2 tsp	**Olive Oil**
2	handfuls **Watercress**
120g	cooked **Puy Lentils**
25g	**Goat's Cheese** (cubed)

Dressing

2 tsp	**Balsamic Vinegar**
½ tsp	**Dijon Mustard**
¼	**Lemon** (juice only)
1 tsp	**Red Wine Vinegar**
2	**Strawberries** (mashed)

Preparation

1. Roast the **beetroot**, **squash**, **parsnip** and **garlic** in 2 tsp **oil** for 30 mins at 180°C.
2. Whisk the **dressing** well.
3. Add the **watercress** to the cooked veg, stir in the **lentils** and dressing, and serve topped with the **cheese**.

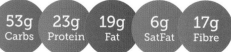

53g	23g	19g	6g	17g
Carbs	Protein	Fat	SatFat	Fibre

Weight | 440g

5	480
5-a-day	Cals

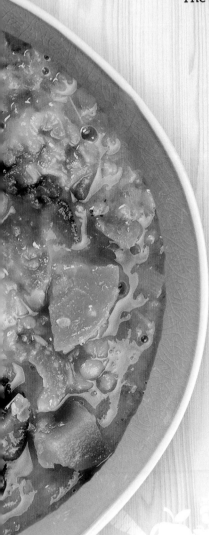

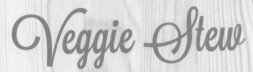

Veggie Stew

The easiest way to get all 5 of your 5-a-day!

Ingredients

80g	**Aubergine** (cubed)
80g	**Butternut Squash** (small cubes)
1	**Carrot** (chopped)
½	**Celery** stalk (sliced)
4	**Cherry Tomatoes** (halved)
1 clove	**Garlic** (minced)
40g	**Leek** (thinly sliced)
30g	dried **Red Split Lentils**
½ tsp	**Smoked Paprika**
1 sprig	**Thyme** (leaves, chopped)
300ml	**Vegetable Stock** (½ cube)
¼	**Yellow Pepper** (sliced)

Preparation

1. Add **all the ingredients** to a slow cooker and cook on medium for 3-4 hours.

215 Cals

5½ 5-a-day

14g Fibre

0g SatFat

3g Fat

12g Protein

38g Carbs

Weight | 480g

Beef & Pearl Barley Stew

A thick stew to warm your cockles
and delight your appetite

Ingredients

300ml	**Beef Stock** (½ cube)
1	**Carrot** (chopped)
½	**Celery** stalk (chopped)
100g	**Chopped Tomatoes** (tinned)
40g	**Mushrooms** (quartered)
¼	**Onion** (sliced)
½	**Parsnip** (chopped)
25g	uncooked **Pearl Barley**
1 sprig	**Rosemary** (leaves, chopped)
70g	**Stewing Beef** (raw, lean, cubed)
1 sprig	**Thyme** (leaves, chopped)
1 tsp	**Worcestershire Sauce**

Preparation

1. Add **all the ingredients** to a slow cooker.
2. Cook on medium for 4-6 hours, until the beef is soft and the pearl barley swollen.

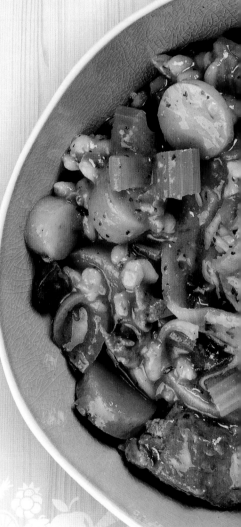

42g	22g	4g	1g	12g
Carbs	Protein	Fat	SatFat	Fibre

Weight | 485g

4	285
5-a-day	Cals

Chicken Tagine

Apricots add zesty sweetness to this lively dish

Ingredients

pinch	**Cinnamon** (ground)
pinch	**Coriander** (ground)
pinch	**Cumin** (ground)
75g	**Chicken Thighs** (raw, skinless, boneless)
40g	**Butternut Squash** (cubed)
1	**Carrot** (chopped)
400ml	**Chicken Stock** (½ cube)
80g	**Chickpeas** (tinned)
100g	**Chopped Tomatoes** (tinned)
3	**Dried Apricots** (chopped)
1 clove	**Garlic** (minced)
⅓	**Red Onion** (chopped)
1 sprig	**Parsley** (large, chopped)

Preparation

1. Rub the **spices** into the **chicken** and pan fry until brown on all sides.
2. Transfer to a slow cooker, adding **all the remaining ingredients** except the parsley.
3. Cook on low for 4 hours.
4. Serve topped with **parsley**.

295 Cals

5½ 5-a-day

13g Fibre

1g SatFat

6g Fat

25g Protein

37g Carbs

Weight | 505g

Vegetable & Bean Chilli

A hearty veggie chilli with sweet potato fingers - perfect for dipping!

Ingredients

40g	**Black Eye Beans** (tinned)
40g	**Butter Beans** (tinned)
1/2	**Carrot** (chopped)
1/2	**Celery** stalk (chopped)
100g	**Chopped Tomatoes** (tinned)
pinch	**Cinnamon** (ground)
pinch	**Coriander** (ground)
pinch	**Cumin** (ground)
1 clove	**Garlic** (minced)
40g	**Kidney Beans** (tinned)
1 tsp	**Olive Oil**
1/4	**Onion** (chopped)
1/2	**Red Chilli** (thinly sliced)
40g	**Sweetcorn** (tinned)
300ml	**Vegetable Stock** (1/2 cube)
100g	**Sweet Potato** (fingers)
40g	**Greek Yogurt**
1 sprig	**Coriander** (large, chopped)

Preparation

1. Add **all the ingredients** (except the sweet potato, yogurt and fresh coriander) to a slow cooker and cook on medium for 4 hours.
2. Later, bake the **sweet potato** in the oven at 180°C for 30 mins (or until golden), turning half way.
3. Serve the sweet potato topped with the bean chilli, **yogurt** and **fresh coriander**.

59g Carbs	16g Protein	10g Fat	3g SatFat	17g Fibre

Weight | 510g

4 1/2 5-a-day

380 Cals

Lamb & Rosemary Stew

After several hours in the slow cooker, the lamb will be ready to melt in your mouth!

Ingredients

1 tsp	**Plain Flour**
75g	**Stewing Lamb** (raw, lean, diced)
1 tsp	**Tomato Purée**
50ml	**Red Wine**
250ml	**Beef Stock** (½ cube)
½	**Carrot** (chopped)
½	**Celery** stalk (chopped)
1 clove	**Garlic** (minced)
¼	**Onion** (thinly sliced)
25g	uncooked **Pearl Barley**
1 sprig	**Rosemary** (leaves, chopped)
80g	**Broccoli** (small florets)
20g	**Cabbage** (sliced)

Preparation

1. Season the **flour** with salt & pepper, then use it to coat the **lamb**.

2. Dry fry the lamb over a medium heat until browned. Transfer to a slow cooker.

3. In the same pan, mix the **tomato purée**, **wine** and **stock**. Bring to the boil.

4. Pour the mixture into the slow cooker. Add the **remaining ingredients** except the cabbage and broccoli. Cook on low for 4-6 hours.

5. When the stew is ready, boil or steam the **broccoli** and **cabbage** for 3 mins, stir through and serve.

405 Cals

3 5-a-day

12g Fibre

5g SatFat

13g Fat

28g Protein

37g Carbs

Weight | 415g

Prawn & Kale Stir-fry

A vibrant Asian taste sensation
that is ready in minutes

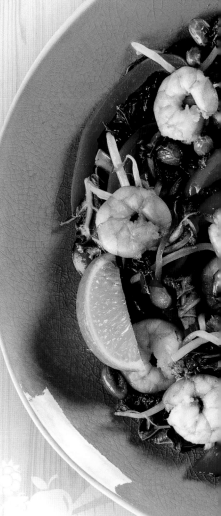

Ingredients

1 tsp	Olive Oil
100g	cooked King Prawns
½	Red Pepper (sliced)
½	Red Chilli (finely chopped)
1 clove	Garlic (minced)
1 inch	Ginger (finely chopped)
80g	cooked Soya Beans
2 tsp	Soy Sauce
2 tsp	Fish Sauce
2 tsp	Mirin
80g	Beansprouts
2	handfuls Kale
1 sprig	Coriander (chopped)
½	Lime (juice only)

Preparation

1. Heat 1 tsp **oil** in a wok until very hot. Fry the **prawns**, **pepper**, **chilli**, **garlic** and **ginger** for 2 mins.

2. Add the **soya beans**, **soy sauce**, **fish sauce** and **mirin**, and heat for another minute.

3. Sprinkle in the **beansprouts** and **kale**, cooking for a further 2 mins.

4. Serve scattered with **coriander** and a squeeze of **lime**.

20g	32g	11g	1g	9g
Carbs	Protein	Fat	SatFat	Fibre

Weight | 280g

3½	325
5-a-day	Cals

Beef & Mushroom Stir-fry

This speedy stir-fry provides 4 of your 5-a-day in record time!

Ingredients

1 tsp	Olive Oil
100g	Beef Sirloin (raw, thin strips)
1 inch	Ginger (finely sliced)
1 clove	Garlic (minced)
40g	Bamboo Shoots
40g	Beansprouts
80g	Mushrooms (sliced)
½	Red Pepper (sliced)
80g	Sugar Snap Peas
2 tbsp	Oyster Sauce
1 tsp	Soy Sauce

Preparation

1. Heat a wok until very hot. Add 1 tsp **oil** and the **beef** strips, cooking for 2 mins.

2. Add the **ginger**, **garlic** and **all of the vegetables**, and fry for a further 2 mins.

3. Stir in the **oyster sauce** and **soy sauce**. Cook for 1 min and serve.

330 Cals

4 5-a-day

6g Fibre

6g SatFat

18g Fat

29g Protein

16g Carbs

Weight | 350g

Tofu & Bean Stir-fry

The chilli bean sauce offers a full-flavoured
jumble for veggie-lovers

Ingredients

1 tsp	**Olive Oil**
1	**Carrot** (sliced)
160g	**Cauliflower** (chopped)
1/3	**Courgette** (batons)
1/3	**Red Onion** (sliced)
100g	**Smoked Tofu** (cubed)
1 clove	**Garlic** (finely sliced)
1 tbsp	**Chilli Bean Sauce**
1 tsp	**Soy Sauce**

Preparation

1. Heat a wok until very
   hot. Add 1 tsp **oil** and
   all of the vegetables,
   frying for 3 mins.

2. Next, mix in the **tofu**,
   garlic, **chilli bean sauce**,
   soy sauce and 2 tbsp water.

3. Cook for a further
   2 mins and serve.

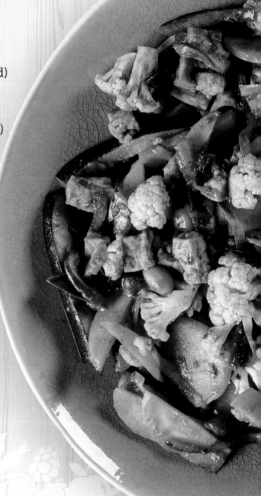

24g Carbs
27g Protein
17g Fat
3g SatFat
8g Fibre

3½ 5-a-day
355 Cals

Weight | 300g

Chicken & Cashew Stir-fry

Our highest-protein dish, popping a whopping 50g!

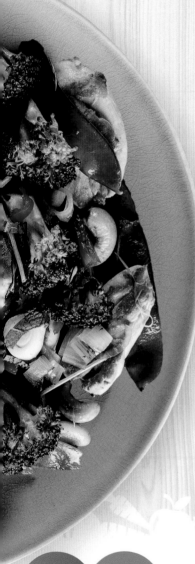

Ingredients

1 tsp	**Olive Oil**
150g	**Chicken Breast** (raw, skinless, sliced)
½	**Red Chilli** (finely sliced)
1 inch	**Ginger** (finely chopped)
2	**Spring Onions** (sliced)
80g	**Mangetout**
1 tbsp	**Cashews**
160g	**Broccoli** (florets, blanched)
2 tsp	**Fish Sauce**
½	**Lemongrass** stalk (finely chopped)
½	**Lime** (juice only)
6	**Thai Basil** leaves (torn)
5	**Mint** leaves (chopped)

Preparation

1. Heat a wok until very hot. Add 1 tsp **oil** and the **chicken** strips.

2. After 2 mins, add the **chilli**, **ginger**, **spring onion**, **mangetout**, **cashews** and **broccoli**. Fry for 3 mins, or until the chicken is cooked.

3. Stir through the **fish sauce**, **lemongrass** and **lime juice**, and cook for a further minute.

4. Top with **Thai basil** and **mint** to serve.

360 Cals

3 5-a-day

10g Fibre

2g SatFat

12g Fat

50g Protein

15g Carbs

Weight | 300g

Veg Noodle Stir-fry

You can't go wrong with a classic nutty combo of cashews, noodles & veggies

Ingredients

50g	uncooked **Wholewheat Noodles**
½	**Red Chilli** (sliced)
1 inch	**Ginger** (finely chopped)
1 clove	**Garlic** (minced)
¼	**Onion** (sliced)
1 tsp	**Olive Oil**
1	**Carrot** (batons)
80g	**Pak Choi** (sliced)
1 tbsp	**Cashews**
40g	**Green Beans** (cooked)
2 tsp	**Fish Sauce**
2 tsp	**Soy Sauce**
1 tsp	**Sesame Oil**
1 sprig	**Coriander** (large, chopped)
½	**Lime** (juice only)

Preparation

1. Cook the **noodles** according to pack instructions, drain and set aside.
2. Meanwhile, fry the **chilli**, **ginger**, **garlic** and **onion** in 1 tsp **olive oil** for 1 minute.
3. Add the **carrot**, **pak choi**, **cashews** and **beans**, and cook for 2 mins.
4. Stir in the noodles, **fish sauce**, **soy sauce**, and 1 tsp **sesame oil**, and heat for a further minute.
5. Mix through the **coriander** and **lime juice**, and serve.

54g Carbs	13g Protein	14g Fat	2g SatFat	10g Fibre

3 5-a-day

390 Cals

Weight | 340g

Tom Yum Soup

A mouth-watering, Asian-inspired, spicy bowlful

Ingredients

½	**Carrot** (thin strips)
40g	**Galangal** (sliced)
1 clove	**Garlic** (finely chopped)
1 inch	**Ginger** (finely chopped)
½	**Lemongrass** stalk (sliced)
¼	**Lime** (juice only)
100g	**Prawns** (raw)
½	**Red Chilli** (finely sliced)
400ml	**Vegetable Stock** (½ cube)
2	**Kaffir Lime Leaves** (torn)

Preparation

1. Bring to the boil **all the ingredients** except the kaffir lime leaves.

2. Add the **kaffir lime leaves** and simmer for 3 mins, or until the prawns are cooked.

3. Serve and enjoy!

130 Cals

1 5-a-day

3g Fibre

0g SatFat

1g Fat

18g Protein

12g Carbs

Weight | 395g

Butternut Squash Soup

Slurp up 3 of your 5-a-day for only 140 calories - the perfect light lunch with plenty of nutrients

Ingredients

240g	**Butternut Squash**	(peeled, cubed)
80g	**Chestnut Mushrooms**	(halved)
½	**Onion**	(chopped)
½	**Red Chilli**	(sliced)
1 sprig	**Rosemary**	(leaves, chopped)
1 sprig	**Thyme**	(leaves, chopped)
400ml	**Vegetable Stock**	(½ cube)

Preparation

1. Combine **all the ingredients** in a pan and bring to the boil.
2. Simmer for 20 mins, until the squash is cooked.
3. Whizz in a blender and serve.

28g Carbs	5g Protein	1g Fat	0g SatFat	8g Fibre	3 5-a-day	140 Cals

Weight | 480g

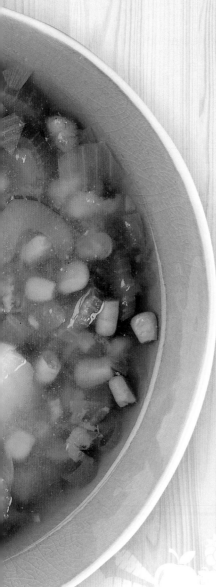

Corn Chowder

This jolly soup is an invigorating mix of sweet and salty

Ingredients

1 sprig **Thyme** (leaves, chopped)
1 **Celery** stalk (finely sliced)
¼ **Onion** (diced)
100g **Potato** (cubed)
1 **Spring Onion** (sliced)
120g **Sweetcorn** (removed from cob)
400ml **Vegetable Stock** (½ cube)

Preparation

1. Add the **thyme** and **all the veg** (except half the sweetcorn) to a pan. Pour in just enough **stock** to cover the veg and bring to the boil.

2. Meanwhile, add the remaining corn to a food processor with 3 tbsp stock and blitz. Add this to the pan.

3. Top up the pan with the remaining veg stock and cook for 15 mins, or until the potatoes are soft.

4. Lightly mash the potato to thicken the chowder, then serve.

190 Cals

2 5-a-day

8g Fibre

0g SatFat

3g Fat

6g Protein

38g Carbs

Weight | 440g

Carrot & Lentil Soup

Chilli & spices give this carrot soup a gentle kick

Ingredients

1 tsp	**Cumin Seeds**
1 tsp	**Olive Oil**
1½	**Carrots** (chopped)
1	**Celery** stalk (chopped)
¼	**Onion** (chopped)
1 clove	**Garlic** (minced)
½	**Red Chilli** (sliced)
30g	dried **Red Split Lentils**
400ml	**Vegetable Stock** (½ cube)
30g	**Greek Yogurt**
1 sprig	**Coriander** (chopped)

Preparation

1. Dry fry the **cumin seeds** in a saucepan until aromatic.

2. Add 1 tsp **oil**, the **vegetables**, **garlic**, **chilli** and **lentils**, and fry for 3 mins.

3. Pour in the **stock**, bring to the boil and simmer for 15 mins, or until the lentils are swollen.

4. Blend until smooth if desired, or leave as a lovely broth.

5. Stir through the **yogurt** and serve topped with **coriander**.

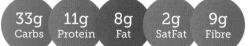

33g	11g	8g	2g	9g
Carbs	Protein	Fat	SatFat	Fibre

Weight | 450g

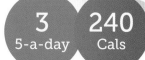

3	240
5-a-day	Cals

Fragrant Crab Soup

This balanced blend of flavours has the
unmistakable taste of Thailand

Ingredients

1 clove **Garlic** (minced)
1 **Spring Onion** (sliced)
½ inch **Ginger** (grated)
1 tsp **Chilli Oil**
¼ **Red Pepper** (thinly sliced)
400ml **Vegetable Stock** (½ cube)
50ml **Coconut Milk** (tinned)
2 **Kaffir Lime Leaves** (torn)
¼ **Lime** (juice & zest)
100g **Crab** (tinned)
1 sprig **Coriander** (large, chopped)
20g **Cabbage** (shredded)
40g **Pak Choi** (chopped)

Preparation

1. Fry the **garlic, spring onion** and
   ginger in 1 tsp **chilli oil** for 3 mins.
2. Add the **pepper** for 3 more mins.
3. Pour in the **stock** and **coconut
   milk**, and bring to the boil.
4. Stir in the **kaffir lime leaves, lime
   juice & zest**. Simmer for 5 mins.
5. Mix through the **crab, coriander,
   cabbage** and **pak choi**.
6. Simmer for 7 mins, then serve.

240 Cals

1½ 5-a-day

4g Fibre

8g SatFat

14g Fat

21g Protein

9g Carbs

Weight | 480g

Black Bean Soup

For those who like a spicy kick, this soup is quick to make and contains 3 types of chilli!

Ingredients

pinch	**Cumin**	(ground)
1 clove	**Garlic**	(minced)
pinch	**Chilli Powder**	
1	**Green Chilli**	(chopped)
1/3	**Red Onion**	(chopped)
1/6	**Courgette**	(chopped)
1 tsp	**Olive Oil**	
1 tsp	**Chipotle Paste**	
400ml	**Vegetable Stock**	(½ cube)
80g	**Black Beans**	(tinned)
40g	**Kidney Beans**	(tinned)
40g	**Sweetcorn**	
1 sprig	**Coriander**	(large, chopped)
1/4	**Lime**	(juice only)
1/4	**Avocado**	(chopped)

Preparation

1. Using a saucepan, fry the **cumin, garlic, chilli powder, chilli, onion** and **courgette** in 1 tsp **oil** for 4 mins.
2. Dissolve the **chipotle paste** in the **stock**.
3. Add the stock, **beans, sweetcorn,** and half of the **coriander** to the saucepan. Bring to the boil and simmer for 5 mins.
4. Squeeze in the **lime juice**, then blend until smooth.
5. Serve topped with **avocado** and the remaining coriander.

20g Carbs	11g Protein	13g Fat	2g SatFat	14g Fibre

3½ 5-a-day

255 Cals

Weight | 450g

Tuscan Tomato Soup

This hearty, wholesome soup contains all 5 of your 5-a-day and over half of your daily fibre needs!

Ingredients

40g	**Leeks** (thinly sliced)
½	**Celery** stalk (chopped)
1	**Carrot** (chopped)
1 clove	**Garlic** (minced)
1 sprig	**Rosemary** (leaves, chopped)
pinch	**Paprika**
1 tsp	**Olive Oil**
200g	**Chopped Tomatoes** (tinned)
500ml	**Vegetable Stock** (½ cube)
80g	**Butter Beans** (tinned)
80g	**Cannellini Beans** (tinned)
1	handful **Kale**

Preparation

1. Fry the **leek, celery, carrot, garlic, rosemary** and **paprika** in 1 tsp **oil** for 10 mins, until the veg softens.

2. Pour in the **tomatoes** and **stock**. Bring to the boil, then simmer for 10 mins.

3. Add the **beans** and bring back to the boil.

4. Finally, add the **kale**, cook for 1 min, then serve.

270 Cals

5 5-a-day

17g Fibre

1g SatFat

7g Fat

15g Protein

39g Carbs

Weight | 650g

Parsnip Cauliflower Soup

Roasting cauliflower unlocks its hidden flavour!

Ingredients

160g	**Cauliflower** (florets)
2	**Parsnips** (cubed)
2 tsp	**Olive Oil**
¼	**Onion** (sliced)
2 cloves	**Garlic** (thinly sliced)
1 sprig	**Thyme** (leaves, chopped)
500ml	**Vegetable Stock** (½ cube)
30g	**Natural Yogurt**

Preparation

1. Coat the **cauliflower** and **parsnip** with 1 tsp **oil** and bake on a tray at 180°C for 20 mins.

2. Meanwhile, gently fry the **onion**, **garlic** and **thyme** in 1 tsp oil for 5 mins, until soft.

3. When the vegetables are cooked, pour the **stock** into the onion and garlic mixture, adding the roasted vegetables. Simmer for 5 mins.

4. Blend until smooth (adding extra water if the soup is too thick).

5. Serve topped with the **yogurt**.

33g Carbs	9g Protein	12g Fat	2g SatFat	12g Fibre		2½ 5-a-day	270 Cals

Weight | 500g

Chicken Noodle Soup

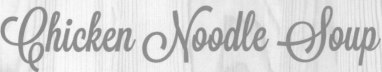

A familiar combination, loaded with flavour - puts a smile on your face every time!

Ingredients

400ml	**Chicken Stock** (½ cube)
1 inch	**Ginger** (grated)
1 clove	**Garlic** (minced)
75g	**Chicken Breast** (raw, skinless, chunks)
50g	dried **Wholewheat Noodles**
40g	**Mushrooms** (sliced)
1	**Spring Onion** (chopped)
40g	**Pak Choi** (chopped)
1 tsp	**Soy Sauce**
1 tsp	**Fish Sauce**
6	**Basil** leaves (torn)

Preparation

1. Heat the **stock** and add the **ginger**, **garlic** and **chicken**. Bring to the boil and simmer for 4 mins.

2. Add the **noodles** and simmer for a further 2 mins.

3. Mix in the **mushrooms**, **onion**, **pak choi** and **soy sauce**. Cook for a further 2 mins.

4. Stir through the **fish sauce** and serve topped with **basil**.

285 Cals

1½ 5-a-day

4g Fibre

0g SatFat

2g Fat

27g Protein

40g Carbs

Weight | 400g

Spring Chicken Soup

This tasty chicken soup packs a whopping 44g protein for under 300 calories!

Ingredients

1 clove	**Garlic** (minced)
⅙	**Red Onion** (sliced)
½	**Carrot** (sliced)
½	**Celery** stalk (sliced)
1 tsp	**Olive Oil**
400ml	**Chicken Stock** (½ cube)
150g	**Chicken Breast** (raw, skinless, sliced)
80g	**Broccoli** (small florets)
20g	**Cabbage** (sliced)
40g	**Peas**
1 sprig	**Parsley** (large, chopped)
1 sprig	**Thyme** (leaves, chopped)

Preparation

1. Fry the **garlic**, **onion**, **carrot** and **celery** in 1 tsp oil, until softened.
2. Pour in the **stock** and **chicken**. Simmer for 8 mins, or until the chicken is cooked through.
3. Stir in the **broccoli** and cook for 2 mins before folding in the **cabbage**, **peas** and **herbs.**
4. Heat for a final 2 mins before serving.

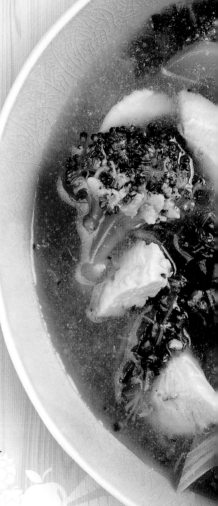

14g Carbs	44g Protein	8g Fat	1g SatFat	9g Fibre

Weight | 550g

3 5-a-day	295 Cals

Acid Raspberry Smoothie

**Our lowest-calorie smoothie
- quench your thirst for only 35 cals**

Ingredients

60g	**Frozen Raspberries**
¼	**Lime** (with skin)
250ml	Water

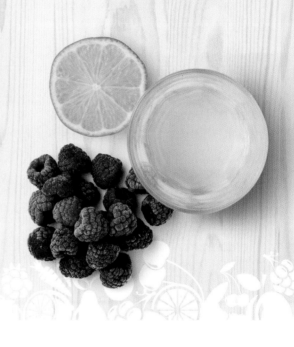

35
Cals

1
5-a-day

4g
Fibre

0g
SatFat

0g
Fat

1g
Protein

7g
Carbs

Weight | 330g

Hey Pesto! Smoothie

This extreme-green, savoury delight
is our lowest-carb smoothie

Ingredients

$1/2$	**Celery** stalk
$1/6$	**Courgette**
$1/8$	**Cucumber**
2	handfuls **Kale**
1	large handful **Lambs Lettuce**
2	handfuls **Spinach**
6	**Basil** leaves
$1/2$	**Lemon** (juice only)
80ml	Water
5	Ice Cubes

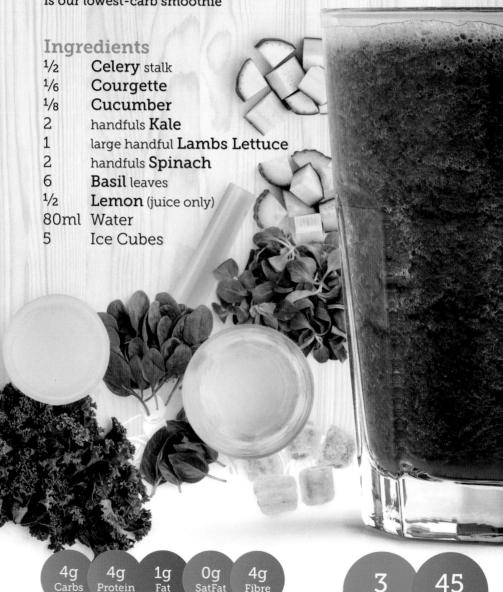

4g Carbs
4g Protein
1g Fat
0g SatFat
4g Fibre

Weight | 395g

3 5-a-day
45 Cals

Carrot Classic Smoothie

This combination is a classic
for a reason: it's delicious!

Ingredients

½	Red Apple
4	Strawberries
½	Carrot
½	Celery stalk
100ml	Water
5	Ice Cubes

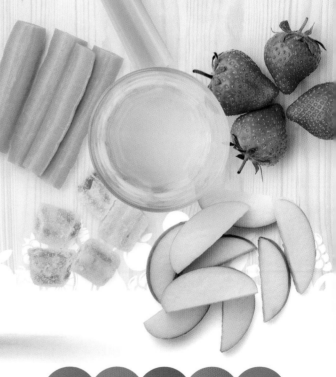

75 Cals

3 5-a-day

5g Fibre

0g SatFat

0g Fat

1g Protein

18g Carbs

Weight | 400g

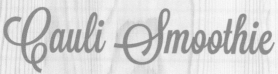

Cauli Smoothie

A surprisingly tasty mix of cauliflower
and apple with a hint of aniseed!

Ingredients

½	Red Apple
80g	Cauliflower
1	Carrot
¼	Cucumber
80g	Fennel
2 inch	Ginger (peeled)
½	Lime (juice only)
140ml	Water
6	Ice Cubes

21g Carbs

4g Protein

1g Fat

0g SatFat

9g Fibre

5 5-a-day

110 Cals

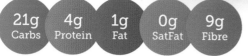

Weight | 630g

Pick up a Pepper Smoothie

This yellow pepper recipe makes
for a savoury, off-beat blitz

Ingredients

½	**Pear** (cored)
¼	**Avocado** (no skin)
½	**Celery** stalk
2	handfuls **Spinach**
¼	**Yellow Pepper** (small)
¼	**Lime** (juice only)
140ml	Water
3	Ice Cubes

125 Cals

3 5-a-day

7g Fibre

1g SatFat

7g Fat

3g Protein

12g Carbs

Weight | 425g

Grass in a Glass Smoothie

Like the smell of freshly-cut grass on a spring morning
(but in a thick, creamy smoothie!)

Ingredients

½	**Pear**	(cored)
1	**Red Apple**	(small)
¼	**Avocado**	(no skin)
2	handfuls **Kale**	
1	sprig **Parsley**	(large)
¼	**Lime**	(juice only)
140ml	Water	
3	Ice Cubes	

25g Carbs

3g Protein

8g Fat

1g SatFat

9g Fibre

3 5-a-day

175 Cals

Weight | 480g

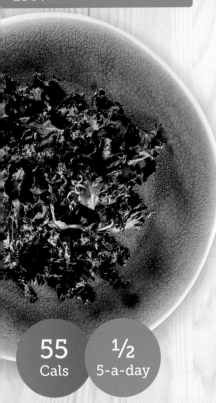

Kale Crisps

Ingredients

2	handfuls	**Kale**
pinch	**Smoked Paprika**	
¼	**Lemon** (juice & zest)	

Preparation

1. Mix the **kale** with 1 tsp **oil**, **paprika** and salt & pepper.
2. Spread out on a baking tray and bake at 150°C for 15 mins.
3. Sprinkle with **lemon juice & zest**, and enjoy!

55 Cals

½ 5-a-day

2g Fibre **1g** SatFat **5g** Fat **2g** Protein **1g** Carbs

Weight | 30g

Rosemary Olives

Ingredients

1 clove	**Garlic** (finely chopped)
¼	**Lemon** (juice & zest)
50g	**Olives** (tinned in brine)
1 sprig	**Rosemary** (leaves, chopped)

Preparation

1. Jumble **everything** together and serve.

60 Cals

1 5-a-day

2g Fibre **1g** SatFat **6g** Fat **1g** Protein **1g** Carbs

Weight | 70g

Olives, Feta & Veg

Ingredients

3	**Cherry Tomatoes** (chopped)
10g	**Feta** (small cubes)
4	**Olives** (small, chopped)
¼	**Lemon** (juice only)
20g	**Baby Corn** (matchsticks)
¼	**Carrot** (matchsticks)

Preparation

1. Mix the **tomatoes, feta, olives** & **lemon juice**.
2. Serve with **corn** and **carrot** on the side.

4g Carbs · **3g** Protein · **4g** Fat · **2g** SatFat · **2g** Fibre

1 5-a-day · **60** Cals

Weight | 110g

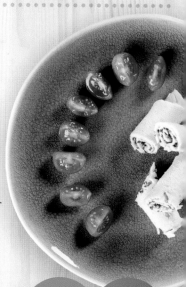

Turkey Rolls

Ingredients

1 tsp	Wholegrain **Mustard**
45g	cooked **Turkey** (sliced)
2	**Cherry Tomatoes** (quartered)

Preparation

1. Spread **mustard** on one side of the **turkey**.
2. Roll into a sausage shape, with the mustard on the inside.
3. Cut in half and serve with the **tomatoes**.

1g Carbs · **11g** Protein · **1g** Fat · **0g** SatFat · **1g** Fibre

0 5-a-day · **65** Cals

Weight | 70g

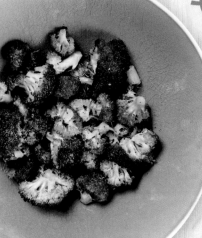

Spiced Broccoli

Ingredients

80g **Broccoli** (florets, chopped)
1 clove **Garlic** (finely sliced)
pinch **Chilli Flakes**
¼ **Lemon** (juice only)

Preparation

1. Heat 1 tsp **oil** on a medium heat and add the **broccoli**, **garlic** and **chilli flakes**.
2. Fry for 5 mins, then serve drizzled with **lemon juice**.

65 Cals

1 5-a-day

3g Fibre | **1g** SatFat | **4g** Fat | **4g** Protein | **3g** Carbs

Weight | 90g

Celery & Nut Butter

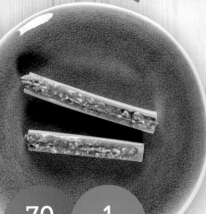

Ingredients

1 **Celery** stalk
2 tsp **Almond Butter**

Preparation

1. Half the **celery** stalk and serve filled with the **almond butter**.

70 Cals

1 5-a-day

2g Fibre | **0g** SatFat | **6g** Fat | **3g** Protein | **1g** Carbs

Weight | 90g

Butterbean Dip

Ingredients

80g	**Butter Beans**	(tinned)
pinch	**Cumin**	(ground)
1 clove	**Garlic**	
¼	**Lemon**	(juice only)
5	**Mint**	leaves
1	**Celery**	stalk (quartered)

Preparation

1. Whizz **all the ingredients** (except the celery) in a food processor. If the consistency is too thick, add a splash of water.
2. Serve with the **celery**.

12g	6g	1g	0g	6g
Carbs	Protein	Fat	SatFat	Fibre

Weight | 180g

2	75
5-a-day	Cals

Lemony Courgette

Ingredients

⅓	**Courgette**	(ribbons)
¼	**Lemon**	(juice only)
½ tsp	**Olive Oil**	
10g	**Parmesan**	(grated)
1 sprig	**Thyme**	(leaves, chopped)

Preparation

1. Mix **all the ingredients** together and enjoy.

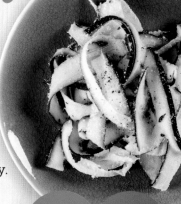

2g	5g	5g	2g	1g
Carbs	Protein	Fat	SatFat	Fibre

Weight | 110g

1	75
5-a-day	Cals

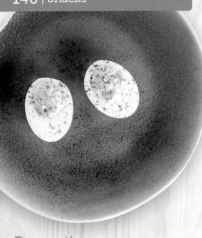

Devilled Eggs

Ingredients

1	**Egg** (hard boiled, peeled)
1 tsp	Mayonnaise
¼ tsp	Dijon Mustard
dash	Tabasco
pinch	Paprika

Preparation

1. Cut the **egg** in half, scoop out the yolk and keep the white to one side.
2. Mash the yolk with the **mayonnaise**, **mustard** and **Tabasco**.
3. Spoon the mixture into the egg white and sprinkle with **paprika**.

95 Cals

0 5-a-day

0g Fibre | **2g** SatFat | **7g** Fat | **8g** Protein | **1g** Carbs

Weight | 65g

Guacamole

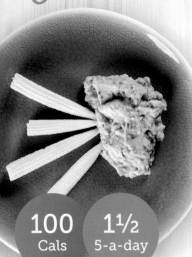

Ingredients

¼	Avocado
pinch	Chilli Flakes
1 sprig	Coriander
¼	**Lime** (juice only)
⅙	Red Onion
40g	**Tomato** (deseeded)
40g	Baby Corn

Preparation

1. Blitz **all the ingredients** except the baby corn in a food processor.
2. Serve with the **baby corn**.

100 Cals

1½ 5-a-day

4g Fibre | **1g** SatFat | **7g** Fat | **2g** Protein | **6g** Carbs

Weight | 150g

Maple Yogurt & Almonds

Ingredients

1 tbsp   Almonds
50g   Natural Yogurt
1 tsp   Maple Syrup

Preparation

1. Toast the **almonds** in a dry frying pan, over a medium heat, until aromatic.

2. Fold the toasted almonds into the **yogurt** and serve drizzled with **maple syrup**.

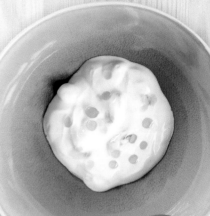

7g Carbs	4g Protein	7g Fat	2g SatFat	1g Fibre

Weight | 65g

0 5-a-day	110 Cals

Yogurt & Seeds

Ingredients

1 tbsp   Mixed Seeds
80g   Natural Yogurt

Preparation

1. Mingle the **seeds** and **yogurt** in a bowl, and enjoy.

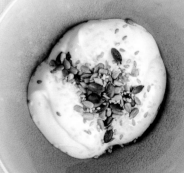

5g Carbs	6g Protein	8g Fat	2g SatFat	1g Fibre

Weight | 90g

0 5-a-day	115 Cals

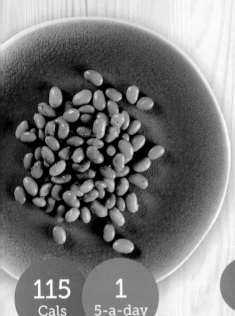

Soya Beans

Ingredients
80g **Soya Beans**

Preparation
1. Boil the **soya beans** in salted water for 2 mins.
2. Serve sprinkled with salt & pepper.

115 Cals

1 5-a-day

4g Fibre

1g SatFat

6g Fat

8g Protein

5g Carbs

Weight | 80g

Spicy Chickpeas

Ingredients
80g   **Chickpeas** (tinned)
pinch **Cumin** (ground)
pinch **Smoked Paprika**

Preparation
1. Combine the **chickpeas** with the **spices**, ½ tsp **olive oil** and salt & pepper.
2. Bake at 180°C for 25 mins, or until the chickpeas are crispy.

115 Cals

1 5-a-day

5g Fibre

1g SatFat

5g Fat

6g Protein

14g Carbs

Weight | 45g

Mixed Nuts

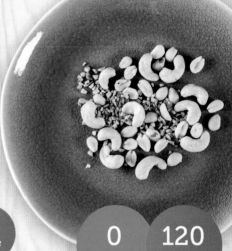

Ingredients

1 tbsp   **Cashews**
½ tbsp   **Peanuts**
½ tbsp   **Hazelnuts** (chopped)

Preparation

1. Toast the **cashews & peanuts** for 4 mins. Serve with the hazelnuts.

3g Carbs	4g Protein	10g Fat	2g SatFat	1g Fibre

0 5-a-day   **120** Cals

Weight | 20g

Roasted Pumpkin Seeds

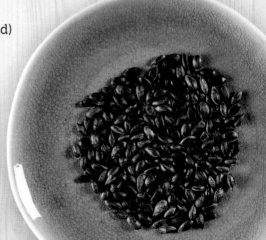

Ingredients

pinch   **Cinnamon** (ground)
pinch   **Nutmeg**
2 tbsp   **Pumpkin Seeds**

Preparation

1. Combine **all the ingredients** and bake at 150°C for 15 mins, stirring half way.

4g Carbs	5g Protein	9g Fat	2g SatFat	2g Fibre

0 5-a-day   **120** Cals

Weight | 15g

Mozzarella & Tomato

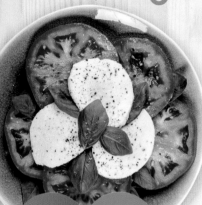

Ingredients

200g **Beef Tomato** (sliced across the core)

40g **Mozzarella** (thickly sliced)

6 **Basil** leaves

Preparation

1. Layer the **tomato**, **mozzarella** and **basil** on a plate and serve.

130 Cals   **1** 5-a-day

2g Fibre   **6g** SatFat   **8g** Fat   **9g** Protein   **6g** Carbs

Weight | 240g

Tuna Lettuce Wraps

Ingredients

70g **Tuna** (tinned)

1 **Spring Onion** (sliced)

2 tsp **Mayonnaise**

2 **Little Gem Lettuce** leaves

Preparation

1. Stir together the **tuna**, **onion** and **mayonnaise**.

2. Spoon the mixture into the **lettuce** leaves and serve.

135 Cals   **½** 5-a-day

1g Fibre   **1g** SatFat   **6g** Fat   **18g** Protein   **2g** Carbs

Weight | 125g

Homemade Beans

Ingredients

⅛	**Onion** (finely chopped)
pinch	**Smoked Paprika**
pinch	**Thyme** (dried)
1 clove	**Garlic** (minced)
½ tsp	**Soy Sauce**
½ tsp	**Honey**
100g	**Chopped Tomatoes** (tinned)
80g	**Cannellini Beans** (tinned)

Preparation

1. Heat ½ tsp **oil** over a low heat. Add the **onion**, **paprika** and **thyme**. Fry gently for 3 mins, then add the **garlic**.

2. Pour in the **soy sauce**, **honey** and **tomatoes**. Bring to the boil and simmer for 2 mins.

3. Stir in the **beans** and cook gently for 5 more mins, or until the sauce has thickened.

21g Carbs	8g Protein	3g Fat	0g SatFat	6g Fibre		2 5-a-day	135 Cals

Weight | 140g

Cheesy Oatcakes

Ingredients

⅛	**Cucumber** (chopped)
50g	**Cottage Cheese**
2	**Oatcakes**

15g Carbs	7g Protein	7g Fat	3g SatFat	2g Fibre		½ 5-a-day	150 Cals

Weight | 110g

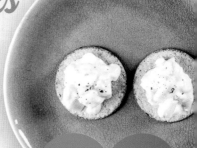

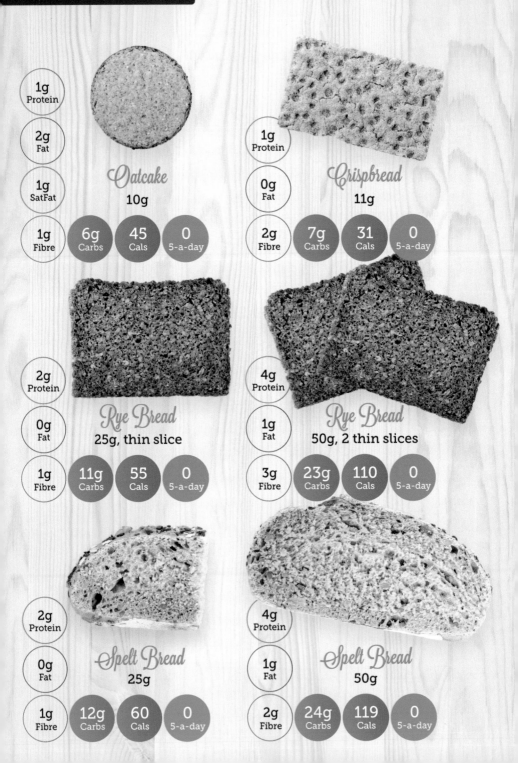

Oatcake
10g

1g Protein
2g Fat
1g SatFat
1g Fibre
6g Carbs
45 Cals
0 5-a-day

Crispbread
11g

1g Protein
0g Fat
2g Fibre
7g Carbs
31 Cals
0 5-a-day

Rye Bread
25g, thin slice

2g Protein
0g Fat
1g Fibre
11g Carbs
55 Cals
0 5-a-day

Rye Bread
50g, 2 thin slices

4g Protein
1g Fat
3g Fibre
23g Carbs
110 Cals
0 5-a-day

Spelt Bread
25g

2g Protein
0g Fat
1g Fibre
12g Carbs
60 Cals
0 5-a-day

Spelt Bread
50g

4g Protein
1g Fat
2g Fibre
24g Carbs
119 Cals
0 5-a-day

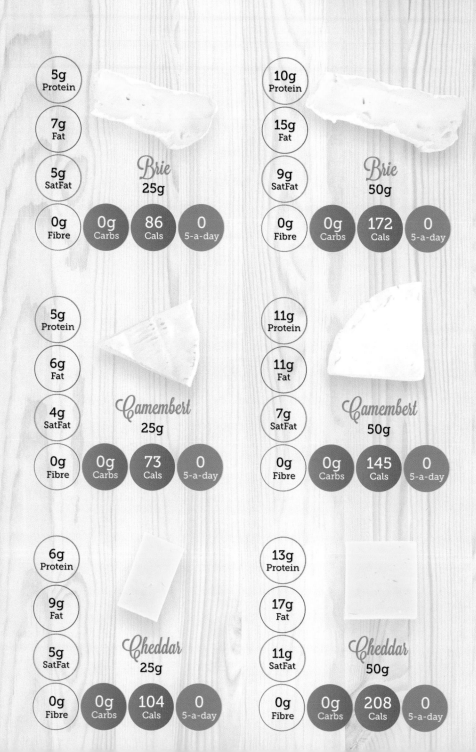

Brie 25g

5g Protein
7g Fat
5g SatFat
0g Fibre
0g Carbs
86 Cals
0 5-a-day

Brie 50g

10g Protein
15g Fat
9g SatFat
0g Fibre
0g Carbs
172 Cals
0 5-a-day

Camembert 25g

5g Protein
6g Fat
4g SatFat
0g Fibre
0g Carbs
73 Cals
0 5-a-day

Camembert 50g

11g Protein
11g Fat
7g SatFat
0g Fibre
0g Carbs
145 Cals
0 5-a-day

Cheddar 25g

6g Protein
9g Fat
5g SatFat
0g Fibre
0g Carbs
104 Cals
0 5-a-day

Cheddar 50g

13g Protein
17g Fat
11g SatFat
0g Fibre
0g Carbs
208 Cals
0 5-a-day

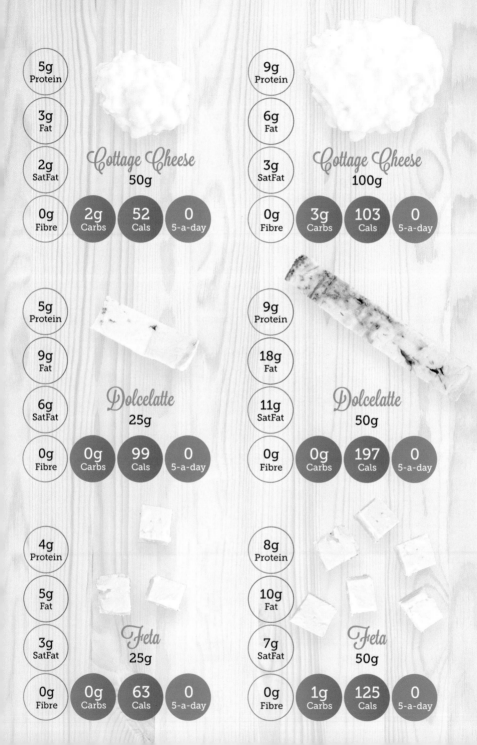

Cottage Cheese
50g

- 5g Protein
- 3g Fat
- 2g SatFat
- 0g Fibre
- 2g Carbs
- 52 Cals
- 0 5-a-day

Cottage Cheese
100g

- 9g Protein
- 6g Fat
- 3g SatFat
- 0g Fibre
- 3g Carbs
- 103 Cals
- 0 5-a-day

Dolcelatte
25g

- 5g Protein
- 9g Fat
- 6g SatFat
- 0g Fibre
- 0g Carbs
- 99 Cals
- 0 5-a-day

Dolcelatte
50g

- 9g Protein
- 18g Fat
- 11g SatFat
- 0g Fibre
- 0g Carbs
- 197 Cals
- 0 5-a-day

Feta
25g

- 4g Protein
- 5g Fat
- 3g SatFat
- 0g Fibre
- 0g Carbs
- 63 Cals
- 0 5-a-day

Feta
50g

- 8g Protein
- 10g Fat
- 7g SatFat
- 0g Fibre
- 1g Carbs
- 125 Cals
- 0 5-a-day

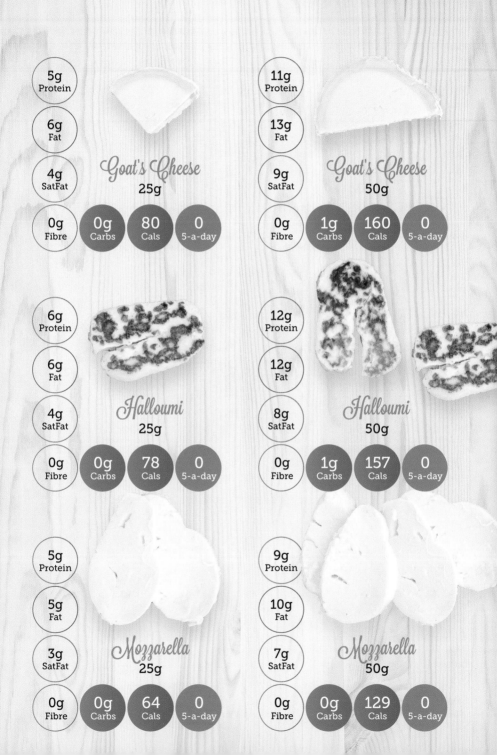

5g Protein
6g Fat
4g SatFat
0g Fibre
Goat's Cheese
25g
0g Carbs
80 Cals
0 5-a-day

11g Protein
13g Fat
9g SatFat
0g Fibre
Goat's Cheese
50g
1g Carbs
160 Cals
0 5-a-day

6g Protein
6g Fat
4g SatFat
0g Fibre
Halloumi
25g
0g Carbs
78 Cals
0 5-a-day

12g Protein
12g Fat
8g SatFat
0g Fibre
Halloumi
50g
1g Carbs
157 Cals
0 5-a-day

5g Protein
5g Fat
3g SatFat
0g Fibre
Mozzarella
25g
0g Carbs
64 Cals
0 5-a-day

9g Protein
10g Fat
7g SatFat
0g Fibre
Mozzarella
50g
0g Carbs
129 Cals
0 5-a-day

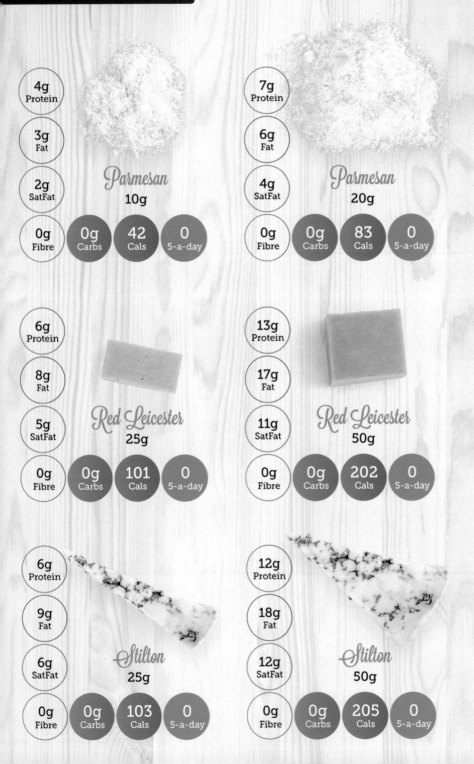

4g
Protein

3g
Fat

2g
SatFat

0g
Fibre

Parmesan
10g

0g
Carbs

42
Cals

0
5-a-day

7g
Protein

6g
Fat

4g
SatFat

0g
Fibre

Parmesan
20g

0g
Carbs

83
Cals

0
5-a-day

6g
Protein

8g
Fat

5g
SatFat

0g
Fibre

Red Leicester
25g

0g
Carbs

101
Cals

0
5-a-day

13g
Protein

17g
Fat

11g
SatFat

0g
Fibre

Red Leicester
50g

0g
Carbs

202
Cals

0
5-a-day

6g
Protein

9g
Fat

6g
SatFat

0g
Fibre

Stilton
25g

0g
Carbs

103
Cals

0
5-a-day

12g
Protein

18g
Fat

12g
SatFat

0g
Fibre

Stilton
50g

0g
Carbs

205
Cals

0
5-a-day

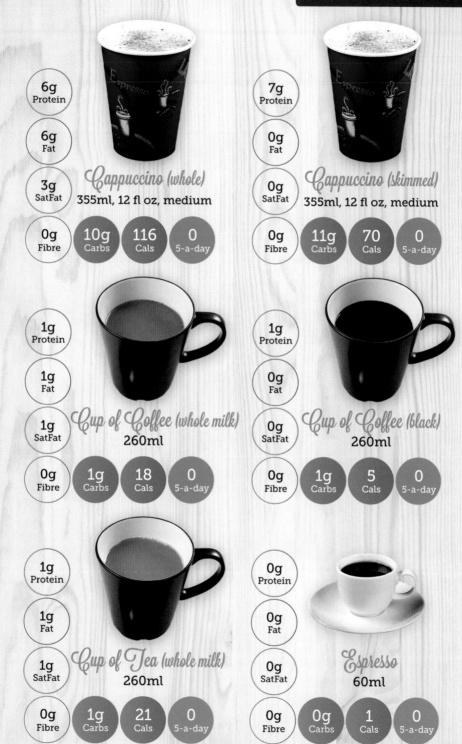

Cappuccino (whole)
355ml, 12 fl oz, medium

6g Protein
6g Fat
3g SatFat
0g Fibre
10g Carbs
116 Cals
0 5-a-day

Cappuccino (skimmed)
355ml, 12 fl oz, medium

7g Protein
0g Fat
0g SatFat
0g Fibre
11g Carbs
70 Cals
0 5-a-day

Cup of Coffee (whole milk)
260ml

1g Protein
1g Fat
1g SatFat
0g Fibre
1g Carbs
18 Cals
0 5-a-day

Cup of Coffee (black)
260ml

1g Protein
0g Fat
0g SatFat
0g Fibre
1g Carbs
5 Cals
0 5-a-day

Cup of Tea (whole milk)
260ml

1g Protein
1g Fat
1g SatFat
0g Fibre
1g Carbs
21 Cals
0 5-a-day

Espresso
60ml

0g Protein
0g Fat
0g SatFat
0g Fibre
0g Carbs
1 Cals
0 5-a-day

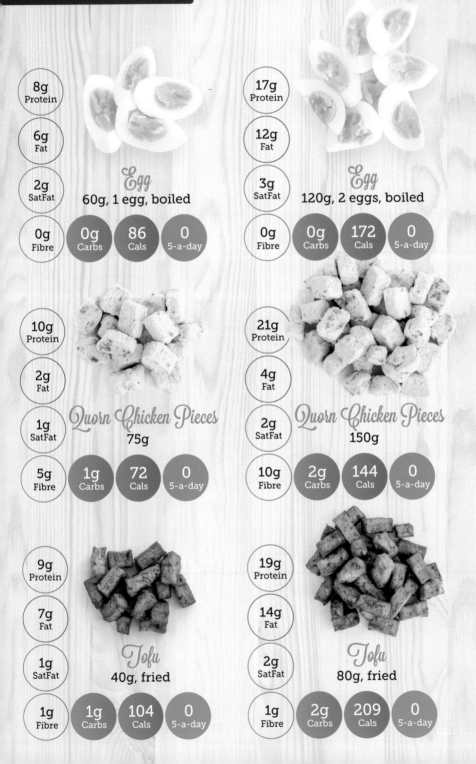

8g Protein
6g Fat
2g SatFat
0g Fibre

Egg
60g, 1 egg, boiled

0g Carbs
86 Cals
0 5-a-day

17g Protein
12g Fat
3g SatFat
0g Fibre

Egg
120g, 2 eggs, boiled

0g Carbs
172 Cals
0 5-a-day

10g Protein
2g Fat
1g SatFat
5g Fibre

Quorn Chicken Pieces
75g

1g Carbs
72 Cals
0 5-a-day

21g Protein
4g Fat
2g SatFat
10g Fibre

Quorn Chicken Pieces
150g

2g Carbs
144 Cals
0 5-a-day

9g Protein
7g Fat
1g SatFat
1g Fibre

Tofu
40g, fried

1g Carbs
104 Cals
0 5-a-day

19g Protein
14g Fat
2g SatFat
1g Fibre

Tofu
80g, fried

2g Carbs
209 Cals
0 5-a-day

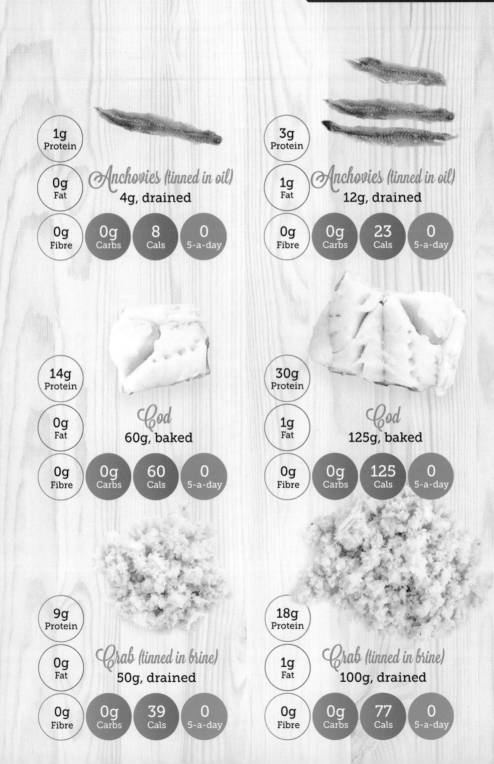

1g Protein

0g Fat

0g Fibre

Anchovies (tinned in oil)
4g, drained

0g Carbs | **8** Cals | **0** 5-a-day

3g Protein

1g Fat

0g Fibre

Anchovies (tinned in oil)
12g, drained

0g Carbs | **23** Cals | **0** 5-a-day

14g Protein

0g Fat

0g Fibre

Cod
60g, baked

0g Carbs | **60** Cals | **0** 5-a-day

30g Protein

1g Fat

0g Fibre

Cod
125g, baked

0g Carbs | **125** Cals | **0** 5-a-day

9g Protein

0g Fat

0g Fibre

Crab (tinned in brine)
50g, drained

0g Carbs | **39** Cals | **0** 5-a-day

18g Protein

1g Fat

0g Fibre

Crab (tinned in brine)
100g, drained

0g Carbs | **77** Cals | **0** 5-a-day

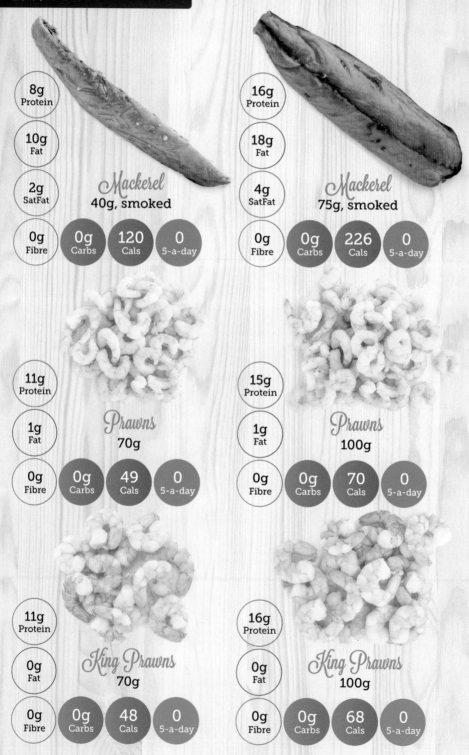

8g Protein
10g Fat
2g SatFat
0g Fibre

Mackerel
40g, smoked

0g Carbs
120 Cals
0 5-a-day

16g Protein
18g Fat
4g SatFat
0g Fibre

Mackerel
75g, smoked

0g Carbs
226 Cals
0 5-a-day

11g Protein
1g Fat
0g Fibre

Prawns
70g

0g Carbs
49 Cals
0 5-a-day

15g Protein
1g Fat
0g Fibre

Prawns
100g

0g Carbs
70 Cals
0 5-a-day

11g Protein
0g Fat
0g Fibre

King Prawns
70g

0g Carbs
48 Cals
0 5-a-day

16g Protein
0g Fat
0g Fibre

King Prawns
100g

0g Carbs
68 Cals
0 5-a-day

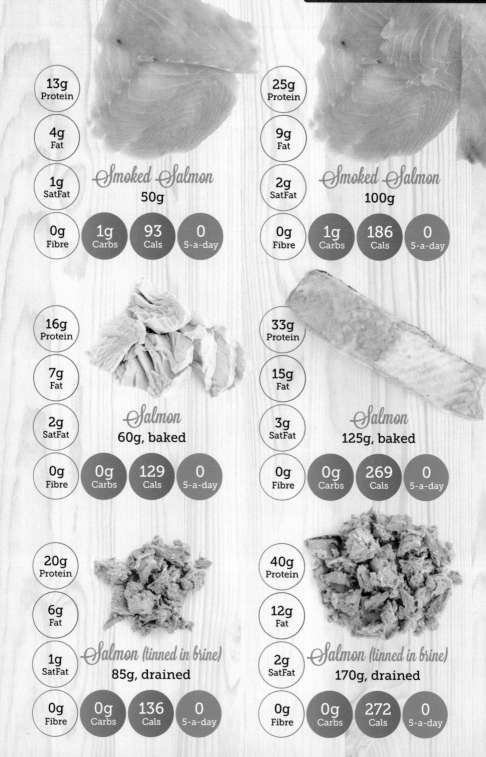

13g Protein
4g Fat
1g SatFat
0g Fibre

Smoked Salmon
50g

1g Carbs
93 Cals
0 5-a-day

25g Protein
9g Fat
2g SatFat
0g Fibre

Smoked Salmon
100g

1g Carbs
186 Cals
0 5-a-day

16g Protein
7g Fat
2g SatFat
0g Fibre

Salmon
60g, baked

0g Carbs
129 Cals
0 5-a-day

33g Protein
15g Fat
3g SatFat
0g Fibre

Salmon
125g, baked

0g Carbs
269 Cals
0 5-a-day

20g Protein
6g Fat
1g SatFat
0g Fibre

Salmon (tinned in brine)
85g, drained

0g Carbs
136 Cals
0 5-a-day

40g Protein
12g Fat
2g SatFat
0g Fibre

Salmon (tinned in brine)
170g, drained

0g Carbs
272 Cals
0 5-a-day

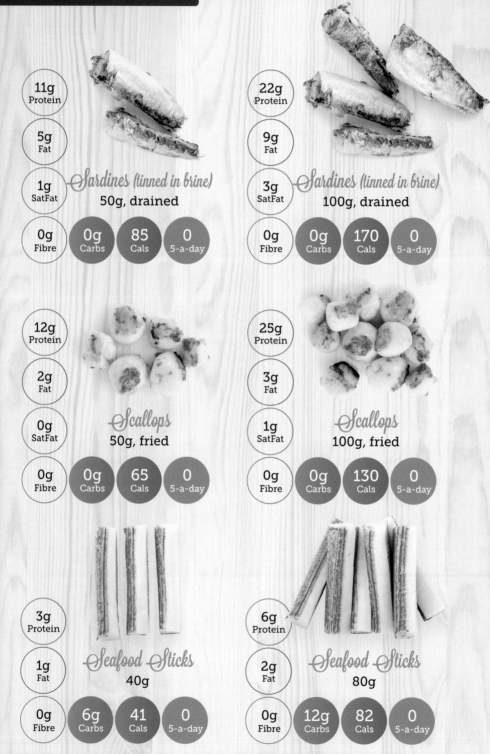

11g Protein
5g Fat
1g SatFat

Sardines (tinned in brine)
50g, drained

0g Fibre
0g Carbs
85 Cals
0 5-a-day

22g Protein
9g Fat
3g SatFat

Sardines (tinned in brine)
100g, drained

0g Fibre
0g Carbs
170 Cals
0 5-a-day

12g Protein
2g Fat
0g SatFat

Scallops
50g, fried

0g Fibre
0g Carbs
65 Cals
0 5-a-day

25g Protein
3g Fat
1g SatFat

Scallops
100g, fried

0g Fibre
0g Carbs
130 Cals
0 5-a-day

3g Protein
1g Fat
0g Fibre

Seafood Sticks
40g

6g Carbs
41 Cals
0 5-a-day

6g Protein
2g Fat
0g Fibre

Seafood Sticks
80g

12g Carbs
82 Cals
0 5-a-day

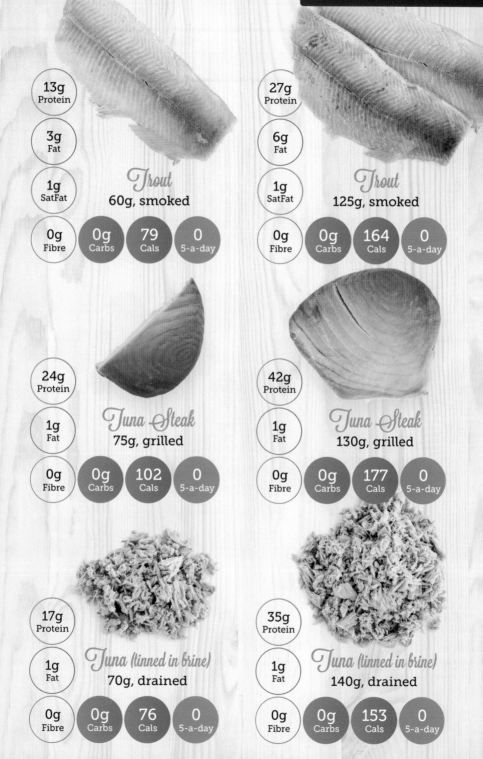

13g
Protein

3g
Fat

1g
SatFat

0g
Fibre

Trout
60g, smoked

0g
Carbs

79
Cals

0
5-a-day

27g
Protein

6g
Fat

1g
SatFat

0g
Fibre

Trout
125g, smoked

0g
Carbs

164
Cals

0
5-a-day

24g
Protein

1g
Fat

0g
Fibre

Tuna Steak
75g, grilled

0g
Carbs

102
Cals

0
5-a-day

42g
Protein

1g
Fat

0g
Fibre

Tuna Steak
130g, grilled

0g
Carbs

177
Cals

0
5-a-day

17g
Protein

1g
Fat

0g
Fibre

Tuna (tinned in brine)
70g, drained

0g
Carbs

76
Cals

0
5-a-day

35g
Protein

1g
Fat

0g
Fibre

Tuna (tinned in brine)
140g, drained

0g
Carbs

153
Cals

0
5-a-day

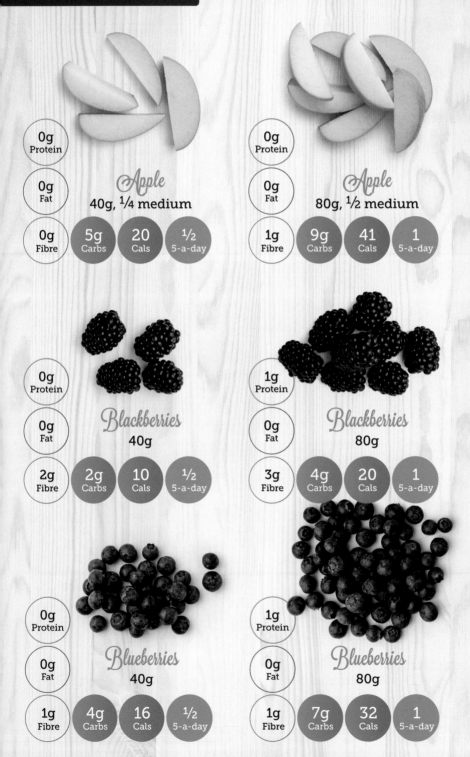

0g Protein

0g Fat

0g Fibre

Apple
40g, ¼ medium

5g Carbs

20 Cals

½ 5-a-day

0g Protein

0g Fat

1g Fibre

Apple
80g, ½ medium

9g Carbs

41 Cals

1 5-a-day

0g Protein

0g Fat

2g Fibre

Blackberries
40g

2g Carbs

10 Cals

½ 5-a-day

1g Protein

0g Fat

3g Fibre

Blackberries
80g

4g Carbs

20 Cals

1 5-a-day

0g Protein

0g Fat

1g Fibre

Blueberries
40g

4g Carbs

16 Cals

½ 5-a-day

1g Protein

0g Fat

1g Fibre

Blueberries
80g

7g Carbs

32 Cals

1 5-a-day

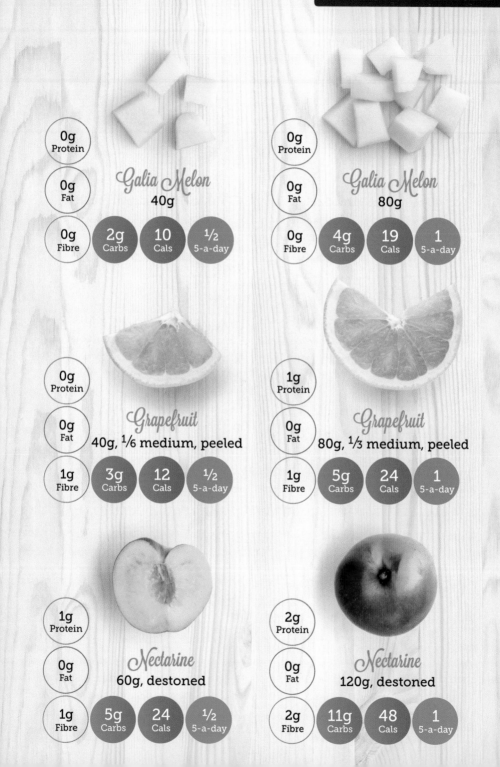

Galia Melon
40g

| 0g Protein | 0g Fat | 0g Fibre | 2g Carbs | 10 Cals | ½ 5-a-day |

Galia Melon
80g

| 0g Protein | 0g Fat | 0g Fibre | 4g Carbs | 19 Cals | 1 5-a-day |

Grapefruit
40g, ⅙ medium, peeled

| 0g Protein | 0g Fat | 1g Fibre | 3g Carbs | 12 Cals | ½ 5-a-day |

Grapefruit
80g, ⅓ medium, peeled

| 1g Protein | 0g Fat | 1g Fibre | 5g Carbs | 24 Cals | 1 5-a-day |

Nectarine
60g, destoned

| 1g Protein | 0g Fat | 1g Fibre | 5g Carbs | 24 Cals | ½ 5-a-day |

Nectarine
120g, destoned

| 2g Protein | 0g Fat | 2g Fibre | 11g Carbs | 48 Cals | 1 5-a-day |

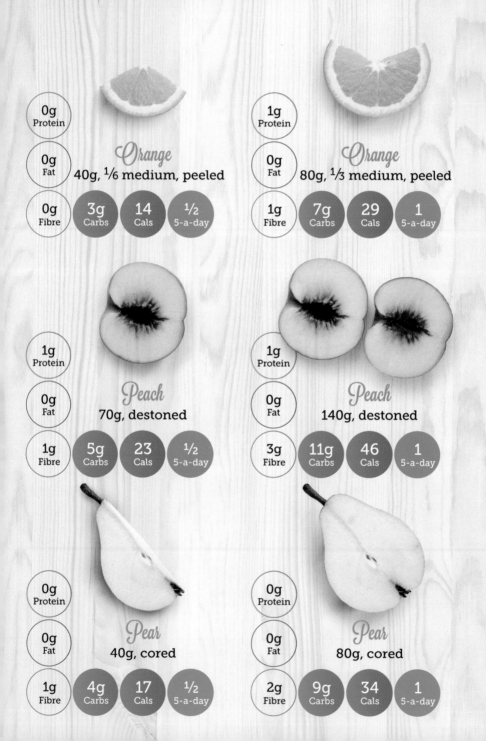

Orange
40g, 1/6 medium, peeled

0g Protein
0g Fat
0g Fibre
3g Carbs
14 Cals
1/2 5-a-day

Orange
80g, 1/3 medium, peeled

1g Protein
0g Fat
1g Fibre
7g Carbs
29 Cals
1 5-a-day

Peach
70g, destoned

1g Protein
0g Fat
1g Fibre
5g Carbs
23 Cals
1/2 5-a-day

Peach
140g, destoned

1g Protein
0g Fat
3g Fibre
11g Carbs
46 Cals
1 5-a-day

Pear
40g, cored

0g Protein
0g Fat
1g Fibre
4g Carbs
17 Cals
1/2 5-a-day

Pear
80g, cored

0g Protein
0g Fat
2g Fibre
9g Carbs
34 Cals
1 5-a-day

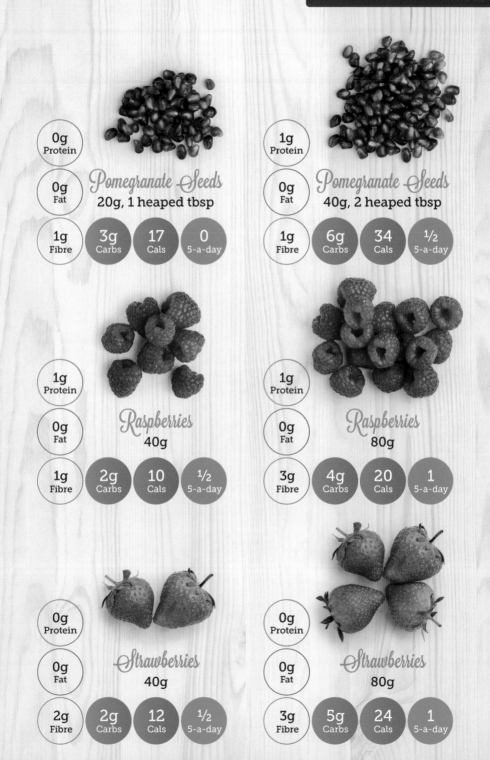

0g
Protein

0g
Fat

1g
Fibre

Pomegranate Seeds
20g, 1 heaped tbsp

3g Carbs
17 Cals
0 5-a-day

1g
Protein

0g
Fat

1g
Fibre

Pomegranate Seeds
40g, 2 heaped tbsp

6g Carbs
34 Cals
½ 5-a-day

1g
Protein

0g
Fat

1g
Fibre

Raspberries
40g

2g Carbs
10 Cals
½ 5-a-day

1g
Protein

0g
Fat

3g
Fibre

Raspberries
80g

4g Carbs
20 Cals
1 5-a-day

0g
Protein

0g
Fat

2g
Fibre

Strawberries
40g

2g Carbs
12 Cals
½ 5-a-day

0g
Protein

0g
Fat

3g
Fibre

Strawberries
80g

5g Carbs
24 Cals
1 5-a-day

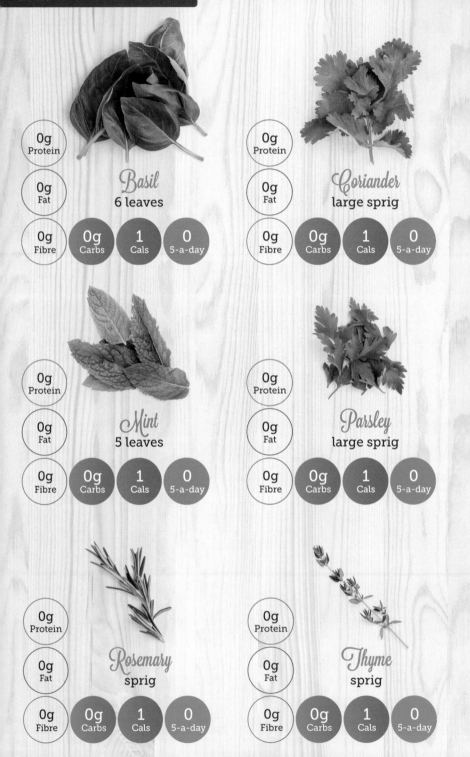

Basil
6 leaves

0g Protein
0g Fat
0g Fibre
0g Carbs
1 Cals
0 5-a-day

Coriander
large sprig

0g Protein
0g Fat
0g Fibre
0g Carbs
1 Cals
0 5-a-day

Mint
5 leaves

0g Protein
0g Fat
0g Fibre
0g Carbs
1 Cals
0 5-a-day

Parsley
large sprig

0g Protein
0g Fat
0g Fibre
0g Carbs
1 Cals
0 5-a-day

Rosemary
sprig

0g Protein
0g Fat
0g Fibre
0g Carbs
1 Cals
0 5-a-day

Thyme
sprig

0g Protein
0g Fat
0g Fibre
0g Carbs
1 Cals
0 5-a-day

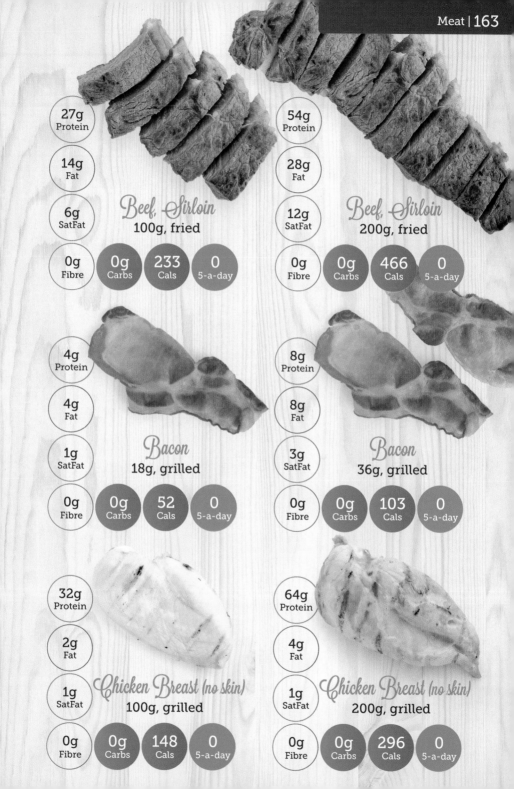

27g Protein
14g Fat
6g SatFat

Beef, Sirloin
100g, fried

0g Fibre | 0g Carbs | 233 Cals | 0 5-a-day

54g Protein
28g Fat
12g SatFat

Beef, Sirloin
200g, fried

0g Fibre | 0g Carbs | 466 Cals | 0 5-a-day

4g Protein
4g Fat
1g SatFat

Bacon
18g, grilled

0g Fibre | 0g Carbs | 52 Cals | 0 5-a-day

8g Protein
8g Fat
3g SatFat

Bacon
36g, grilled

0g Fibre | 0g Carbs | 103 Cals | 0 5-a-day

32g Protein
2g Fat
1g SatFat

Chicken Breast (no skin)
100g, grilled

0g Fibre | 0g Carbs | 148 Cals | 0 5-a-day

64g Protein
4g Fat
1g SatFat

Chicken Breast (no skin)
200g, grilled

0g Fibre | 0g Carbs | 296 Cals | 0 5-a-day

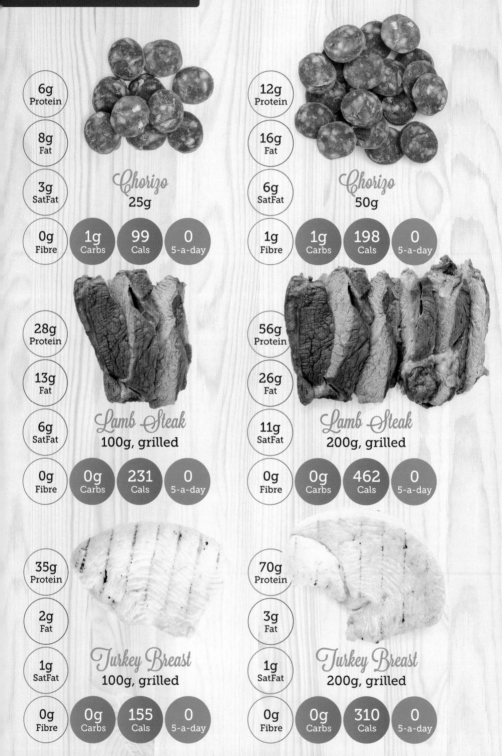

Chorizo
25g

- 6g Protein
- 8g Fat
- 3g SatFat
- 0g Fibre
- 1g Carbs
- 99 Cals
- 0 5-a-day

Chorizo
50g

- 12g Protein
- 16g Fat
- 6g SatFat
- 1g Fibre
- 1g Carbs
- 198 Cals
- 0 5-a-day

Lamb Steak
100g, grilled

- 28g Protein
- 13g Fat
- 6g SatFat
- 0g Fibre
- 0g Carbs
- 231 Cals
- 0 5-a-day

Lamb Steak
200g, grilled

- 56g Protein
- 26g Fat
- 11g SatFat
- 0g Fibre
- 0g Carbs
- 462 Cals
- 0 5-a-day

Turkey Breast
100g, grilled

- 35g Protein
- 2g Fat
- 1g SatFat
- 0g Fibre
- 0g Carbs
- 155 Cals
- 0 5-a-day

Turkey Breast
200g, grilled

- 70g Protein
- 3g Fat
- 1g SatFat
- 0g Fibre
- 0g Carbs
- 310 Cals
- 0 5-a-day

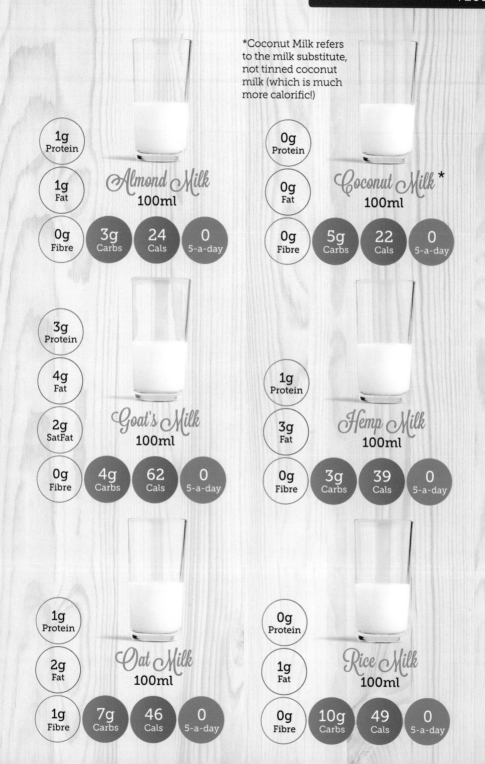

*Coconut Milk refers to the milk substitute, not tinned coconut milk (which is much more calorific!)

Almond Milk
100ml

1g Protein
1g Fat
0g Fibre
3g Carbs
24 Cals
0 5-a-day

Coconut Milk *
100ml

0g Protein
0g Fat
0g Fibre
5g Carbs
22 Cals
0 5-a-day

Goat's Milk
100ml

3g Protein
4g Fat
2g SatFat
0g Fibre
4g Carbs
62 Cals
0 5-a-day

Hemp Milk
100ml

1g Protein
3g Fat
0g Fibre
3g Carbs
39 Cals
0 5-a-day

Oat Milk
100ml

1g Protein
2g Fat
1g Fibre
7g Carbs
46 Cals
0 5-a-day

Rice Milk
100ml

0g Protein
1g Fat
0g Fibre
10g Carbs
49 Cals
0 5-a-day

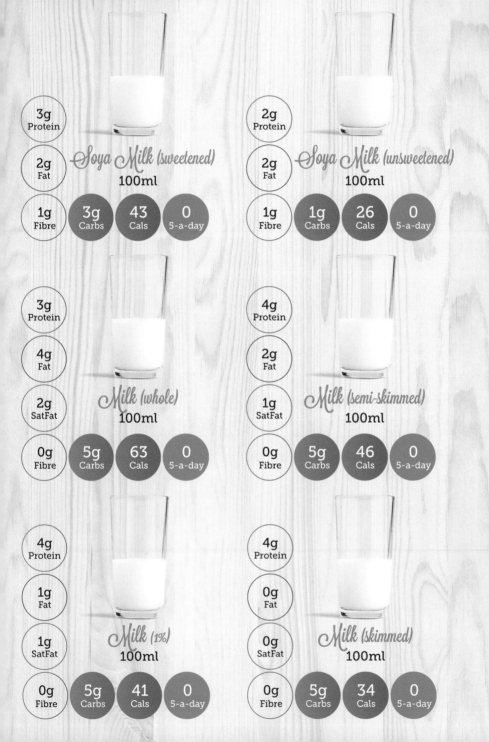

Soya Milk (sweetened)
100ml

3g Protein
2g Fat
1g Fibre
3g Carbs
43 Cals
0 5-a-day

Soya Milk (unsweetened)
100ml

2g Protein
2g Fat
1g Fibre
1g Carbs
26 Cals
0 5-a-day

Milk (whole)
100ml

3g Protein
4g Fat
2g SatFat
0g Fibre
5g Carbs
63 Cals
0 5-a-day

Milk (semi-skimmed)
100ml

4g Protein
2g Fat
1g SatFat
0g Fibre
5g Carbs
46 Cals
0 5-a-day

Milk (1%)
100ml

4g Protein
1g Fat
1g SatFat
0g Fibre
5g Carbs
41 Cals
0 5-a-day

Milk (skimmed)
100ml

4g Protein
0g Fat
0g SatFat
0g Fibre
5g Carbs
34 Cals
0 5-a-day

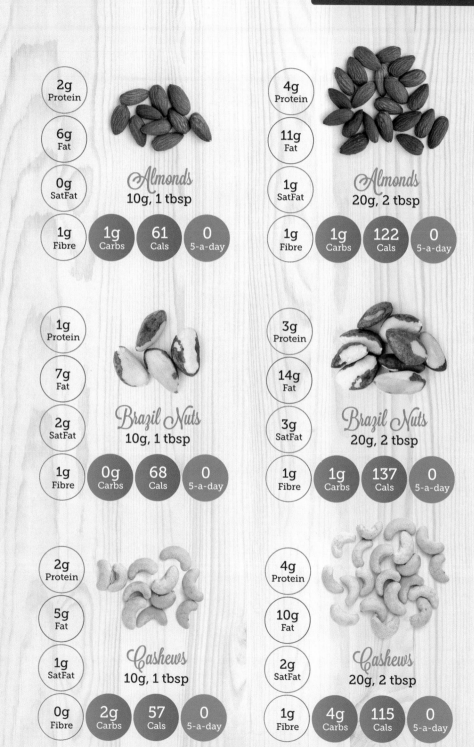

Almonds
10g, 1 tbsp

2g Protein
6g Fat
0g SatFat
1g Fibre
1g Carbs
61 Cals
0 5-a-day

Almonds
20g, 2 tbsp

4g Protein
11g Fat
1g SatFat
1g Fibre
1g Carbs
122 Cals
0 5-a-day

Brazil Nuts
10g, 1 tbsp

1g Protein
7g Fat
2g SatFat
1g Fibre
0g Carbs
68 Cals
0 5-a-day

Brazil Nuts
20g, 2 tbsp

3g Protein
14g Fat
3g SatFat
1g Fibre
1g Carbs
137 Cals
0 5-a-day

Cashews
10g, 1 tbsp

2g Protein
5g Fat
1g SatFat
0g Fibre
2g Carbs
57 Cals
0 5-a-day

Cashews
20g, 2 tbsp

4g Protein
10g Fat
2g SatFat
1g Fibre
4g Carbs
115 Cals
0 5-a-day

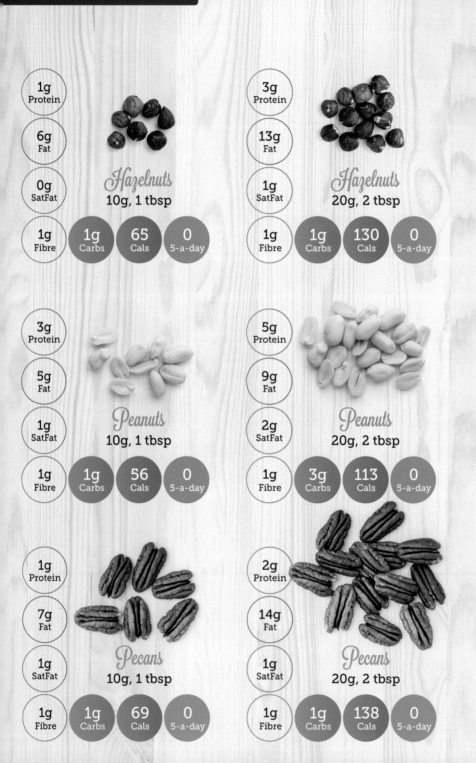

1g Protein
6g Fat
0g SatFat
1g Fibre

Hazelnuts
10g, 1 tbsp

1g Carbs
65 Cals
0 5-a-day

3g Protein
13g Fat
1g SatFat
1g Fibre

Hazelnuts
20g, 2 tbsp

1g Carbs
130 Cals
0 5-a-day

3g Protein
5g Fat
1g SatFat
1g Fibre

Peanuts
10g, 1 tbsp

1g Carbs
56 Cals
0 5-a-day

5g Protein
9g Fat
2g SatFat
1g Fibre

Peanuts
20g, 2 tbsp

3g Carbs
113 Cals
0 5-a-day

1g Protein
7g Fat
1g SatFat
1g Fibre

Pecans
10g, 1 tbsp

1g Carbs
69 Cals
0 5-a-day

2g Protein
14g Fat
1g SatFat
1g Fibre

Pecans
20g, 2 tbsp

1g Carbs
138 Cals
0 5-a-day

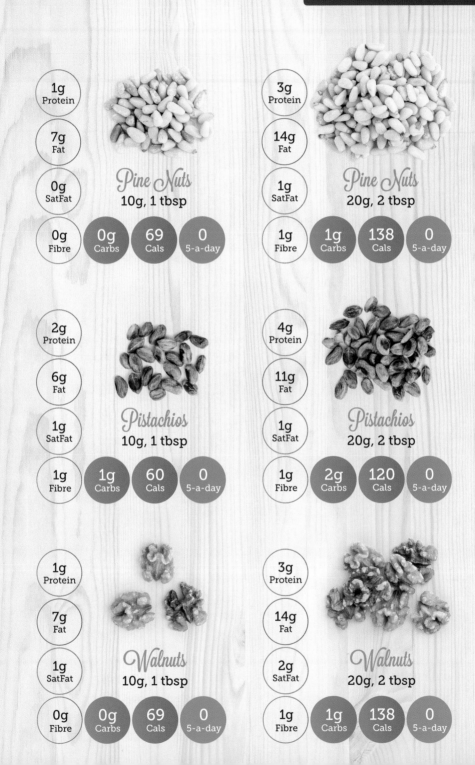

1g Protein
7g Fat
0g SatFat
0g Fibre

Pine Nuts
10g, 1 tbsp

0g Carbs
69 Cals
0 5-a-day

3g Protein
14g Fat
1g SatFat
1g Fibre

Pine Nuts
20g, 2 tbsp

1g Carbs
138 Cals
0 5-a-day

2g Protein
6g Fat
1g SatFat
1g Fibre

Pistachios
10g, 1 tbsp

1g Carbs
60 Cals
0 5-a-day

4g Protein
11g Fat
1g SatFat
1g Fibre

Pistachios
20g, 2 tbsp

2g Carbs
120 Cals
0 5-a-day

1g Protein
7g Fat
1g SatFat
0g Fibre

Walnuts
10g, 1 tbsp

0g Carbs
69 Cals
0 5-a-day

3g Protein
14g Fat
2g SatFat
1g Fibre

Walnuts
20g, 2 tbsp

1g Carbs
138 Cals
0 5-a-day

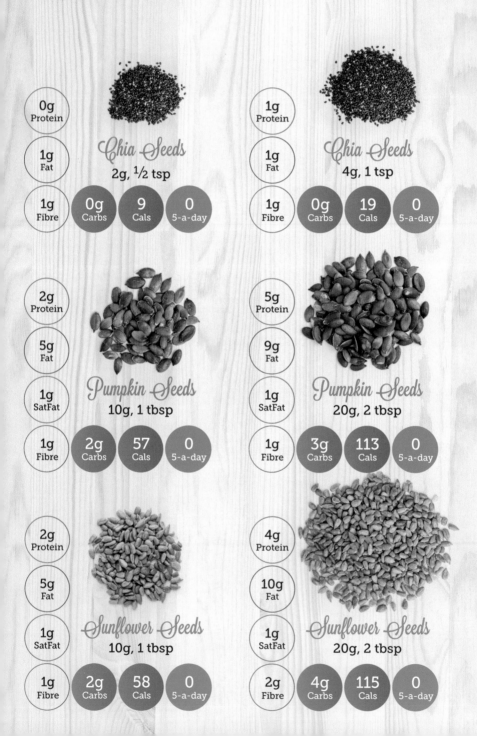

Chia Seeds
2g, ½ tsp

0g Protein
1g Fat
1g Fibre
0g Carbs
9 Cals
0 5-a-day

Chia Seeds
4g, 1 tsp

1g Protein
1g Fat
1g Fibre
0g Carbs
19 Cals
0 5-a-day

Pumpkin Seeds
10g, 1 tbsp

2g Protein
5g Fat
1g SatFat
1g Fibre
2g Carbs
57 Cals
0 5-a-day

Pumpkin Seeds
20g, 2 tbsp

5g Protein
9g Fat
1g SatFat
1g Fibre
3g Carbs
113 Cals
0 5-a-day

Sunflower Seeds
10g, 1 tbsp

2g Protein
5g Fat
1g SatFat
1g Fibre
2g Carbs
58 Cals
0 5-a-day

Sunflower Seeds
20g, 2 tbsp

4g Protein
10g Fat
1g SatFat
2g Fibre
4g Carbs
115 Cals
0 5-a-day

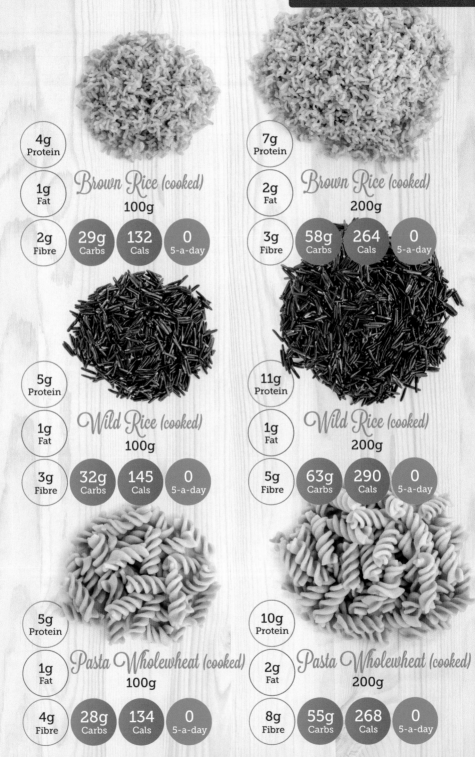

4g Protein

1g Fat

2g Fibre

Brown Rice (cooked)
100g

29g Carbs | 132 Cals | 0 5-a-day

7g Protein

2g Fat

3g Fibre

Brown Rice (cooked)
200g

58g Carbs | 264 Cals | 0 5-a-day

5g Protein

1g Fat

3g Fibre

Wild Rice (cooked)
100g

32g Carbs | 145 Cals | 0 5-a-day

11g Protein

1g Fat

5g Fibre

Wild Rice (cooked)
200g

63g Carbs | 290 Cals | 0 5-a-day

5g Protein

1g Fat

4g Fibre

Pasta Wholewheat (cooked)
100g

28g Carbs | 134 Cals | 0 5-a-day

10g Protein

2g Fat

8g Fibre

Pasta Wholewheat (cooked)
200g

55g Carbs | 268 Cals | 0 5-a-day

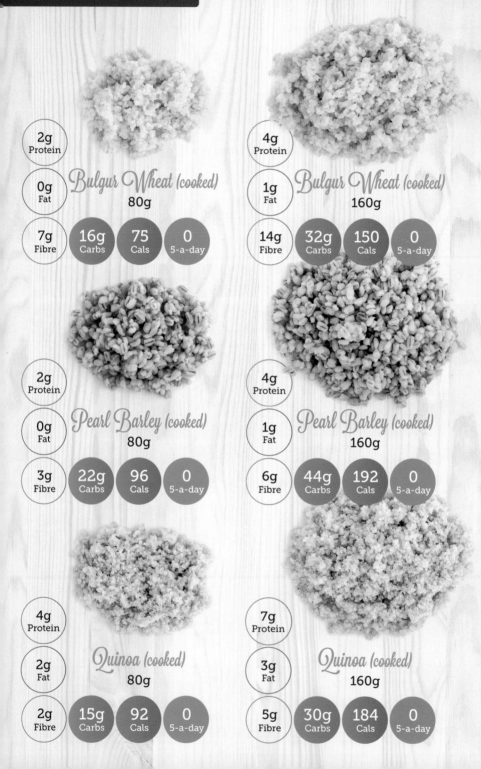

2g
Protein

0g
Fat

7g
Fibre

Bulgur Wheat (cooked)
80g

16g
Carbs

75
Cals

0
5-a-day

4g
Protein

1g
Fat

14g
Fibre

Bulgur Wheat (cooked)
160g

32g
Carbs

150
Cals

0
5-a-day

2g
Protein

0g
Fat

3g
Fibre

Pearl Barley (cooked)
80g

22g
Carbs

96
Cals

0
5-a-day

4g
Protein

1g
Fat

6g
Fibre

Pearl Barley (cooked)
160g

44g
Carbs

192
Cals

0
5-a-day

4g
Protein

2g
Fat

2g
Fibre

Quinoa (cooked)
80g

15g
Carbs

92
Cals

0
5-a-day

7g
Protein

3g
Fat

5g
Fibre

Quinoa (cooked)
160g

30g
Carbs

184
Cals

0
5-a-day

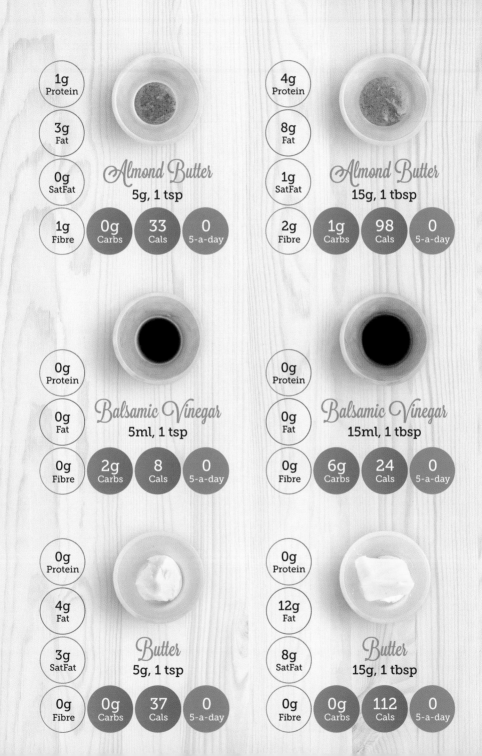

1g Protein
3g Fat
0g SatFat
1g Fibre

Almond Butter
5g, 1 tsp

0g Carbs
33 Cals
0 5-a-day

4g Protein
8g Fat
1g SatFat
2g Fibre

Almond Butter
15g, 1 tbsp

1g Carbs
98 Cals
0 5-a-day

0g Protein
0g Fat
0g Fibre

Balsamic Vinegar
5ml, 1 tsp

2g Carbs
8 Cals
0 5-a-day

0g Protein
0g Fat
0g Fibre

Balsamic Vinegar
15ml, 1 tbsp

6g Carbs
24 Cals
0 5-a-day

0g Protein
4g Fat
3g SatFat
0g Fibre

Butter
5g, 1 tsp

0g Carbs
37 Cals
0 5-a-day

0g Protein
12g Fat
8g SatFat
0g Fibre

Butter
15g, 1 tbsp

0g Carbs
112 Cals
0 5-a-day

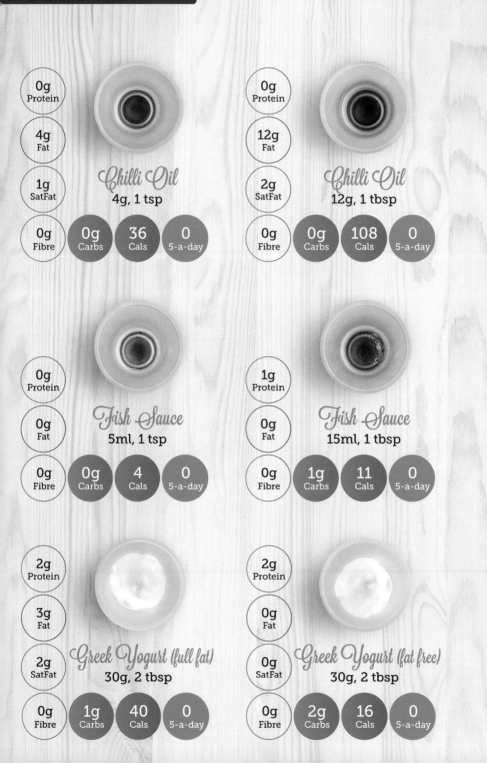

0g
Protein

4g
Fat

1g
SatFat

0g
Fibre

Chilli Oil
4g, 1 tsp

0g
Carbs

36
Cals

0
5-a-day

0g
Protein

12g
Fat

2g
SatFat

0g
Fibre

Chilli Oil
12g, 1 tbsp

0g
Carbs

108
Cals

0
5-a-day

0g
Protein

0g
Fat

0g
Fibre

Fish Sauce
5ml, 1 tsp

0g
Carbs

4
Cals

0
5-a-day

1g
Protein

0g
Fat

0g
Fibre

Fish Sauce
15ml, 1 tbsp

1g
Carbs

11
Cals

0
5-a-day

2g
Protein

3g
Fat

2g
SatFat

0g
Fibre

Greek Yogurt (full fat)
30g, 2 tbsp

1g
Carbs

40
Cals

0
5-a-day

2g
Protein

0g
Fat

0g
SatFat

0g
Fibre

Greek Yogurt (fat free)
30g, 2 tbsp

2g
Carbs

16
Cals

0
5-a-day

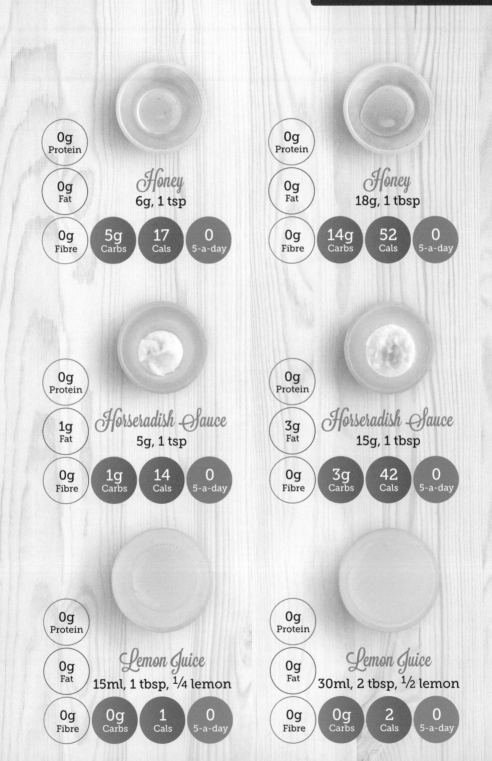

0g Protein
0g Fat
0g Fibre

Honey
6g, 1 tsp

5g Carbs | 17 Cals | 0 5-a-day

0g Protein
0g Fat
0g Fibre

Honey
18g, 1 tbsp

14g Carbs | 52 Cals | 0 5-a-day

0g Protein
1g Fat
0g Fibre

Horseradish Sauce
5g, 1 tsp

1g Carbs | 14 Cals | 0 5-a-day

0g Protein
3g Fat
0g Fibre

Horseradish Sauce
15g, 1 tbsp

3g Carbs | 42 Cals | 0 5-a-day

0g Protein
0g Fat
0g Fibre

Lemon Juice
15ml, 1 tbsp, ¼ lemon

0g Carbs | 1 Cals | 0 5-a-day

0g Protein
0g Fat
0g Fibre

Lemon Juice
30ml, 2 tbsp, ½ lemon

0g Carbs | 2 Cals | 0 5-a-day

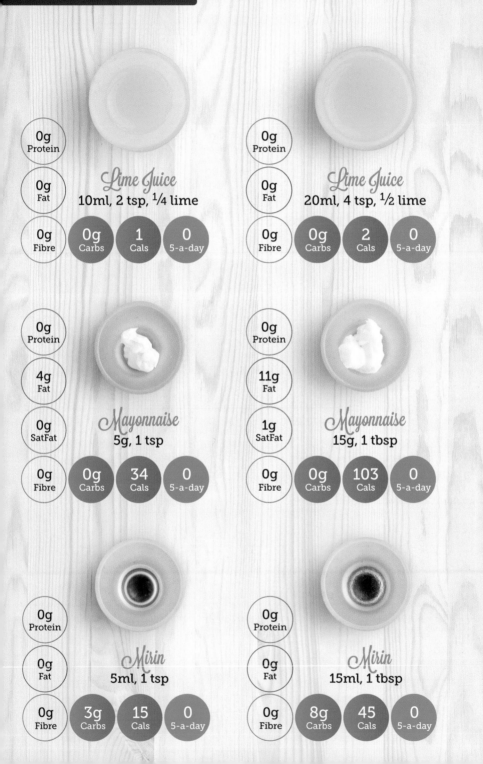

0g
Protein

0g
Fat

0g
Fibre

Lime Juice
10ml, 2 tsp, ¼ lime

0g
Carbs

1
Cals

0
5-a-day

0g
Protein

0g
Fat

0g
Fibre

Lime Juice
20ml, 4 tsp, ½ lime

0g
Carbs

2
Cals

0
5-a-day

0g
Protein

4g
Fat

0g
SatFat

0g
Fibre

Mayonnaise
5g, 1 tsp

0g
Carbs

34
Cals

0
5-a-day

0g
Protein

11g
Fat

1g
SatFat

0g
Fibre

Mayonnaise
15g, 1 tbsp

0g
Carbs

103
Cals

0
5-a-day

0g
Protein

0g
Fat

0g
Fibre

Mirin
5ml, 1 tsp

3g
Carbs

15
Cals

0
5-a-day

0g
Protein

0g
Fat

0g
Fibre

Mirin
15ml, 1 tbsp

8g
Carbs

45
Cals

0
5-a-day

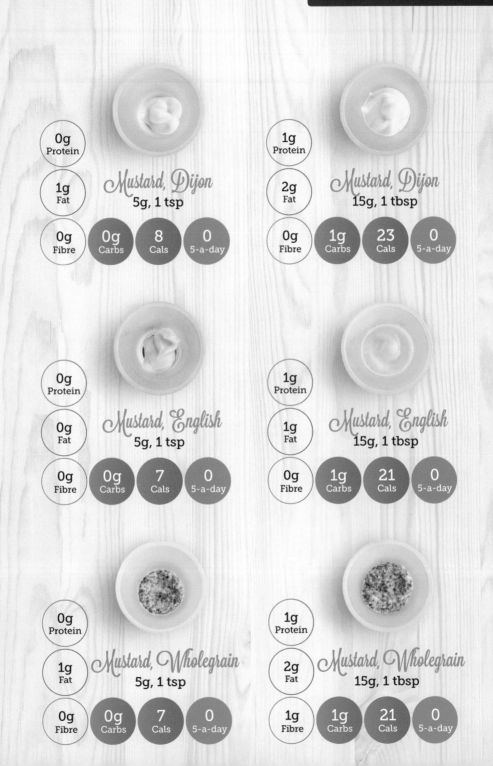

Mustard, Dijon
5g, 1 tsp

0g Protein
1g Fat
0g Fibre
0g Carbs
8 Cals
0 5-a-day

Mustard, Dijon
15g, 1 tbsp

1g Protein
2g Fat
0g Fibre
1g Carbs
23 Cals
0 5-a-day

Mustard, English
5g, 1 tsp

0g Protein
0g Fat
0g Fibre
0g Carbs
7 Cals
0 5-a-day

Mustard, English
15g, 1 tbsp

1g Protein
1g Fat
0g Fibre
1g Carbs
21 Cals
0 5-a-day

Mustard, Wholegrain
5g, 1 tsp

0g Protein
1g Fat
0g Fibre
0g Carbs
7 Cals
0 5-a-day

Mustard, Wholegrain
15g, 1 tbsp

1g Protein
2g Fat
1g Fibre
1g Carbs
21 Cals
0 5-a-day

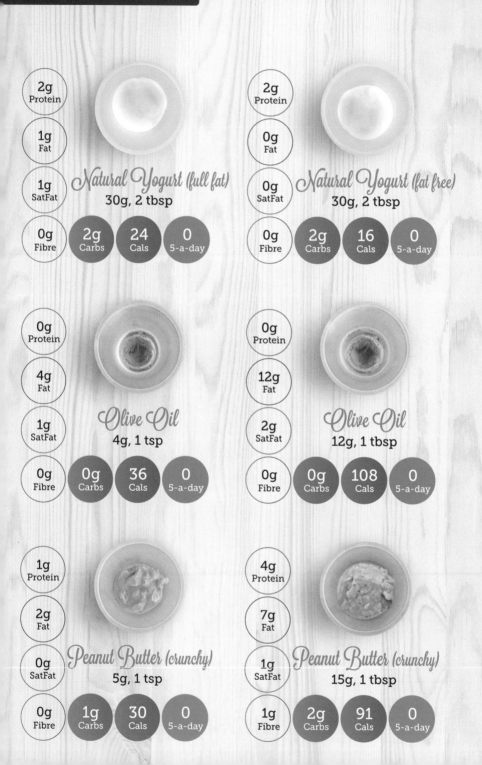

2g Protein
1g Fat
1g SatFat
0g Fibre

Natural Yogurt (full fat)
30g, 2 tbsp

2g Carbs | 24 Cals | 0 5-a-day

2g Protein
0g Fat
0g SatFat
0g Fibre

Natural Yogurt (fat free)
30g, 2 tbsp

2g Carbs | 16 Cals | 0 5-a-day

0g Protein
4g Fat
1g SatFat
0g Fibre

Olive Oil
4g, 1 tsp

0g Carbs | 36 Cals | 0 5-a-day

0g Protein
12g Fat
2g SatFat
0g Fibre

Olive Oil
12g, 1 tbsp

0g Carbs | 108 Cals | 0 5-a-day

1g Protein
2g Fat
0g SatFat
0g Fibre

Peanut Butter (crunchy)
5g, 1 tsp

1g Carbs | 30 Cals | 0 5-a-day

4g Protein
7g Fat
1g SatFat
1g Fibre

Peanut Butter (crunchy)
15g, 1 tbsp

2g Carbs | 91 Cals | 0 5-a-day

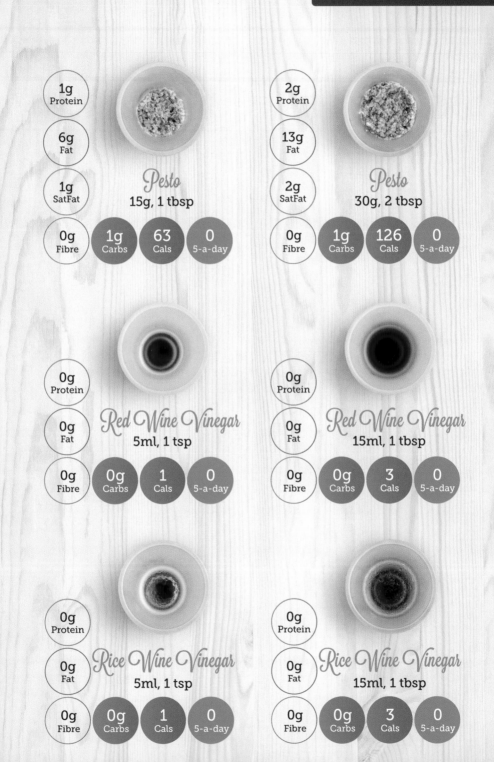

1g Protein
6g Fat
1g SatFat
0g Fibre

Pesto
15g, 1 tbsp

1g Carbs | 63 Cals | 0 5-a-day

2g Protein
13g Fat
2g SatFat
0g Fibre

Pesto
30g, 2 tbsp

1g Carbs | 126 Cals | 0 5-a-day

0g Protein
0g Fat
0g Fibre

Red Wine Vinegar
5ml, 1 tsp

0g Carbs | 1 Cals | 0 5-a-day

0g Protein
0g Fat
0g Fibre

Red Wine Vinegar
15ml, 1 tbsp

0g Carbs | 3 Cals | 0 5-a-day

0g Protein
0g Fat
0g Fibre

Rice Wine Vinegar
5ml, 1 tsp

0g Carbs | 1 Cals | 0 5-a-day

0g Protein
0g Fat
0g Fibre

Rice Wine Vinegar
15ml, 1 tbsp

0g Carbs | 3 Cals | 0 5-a-day

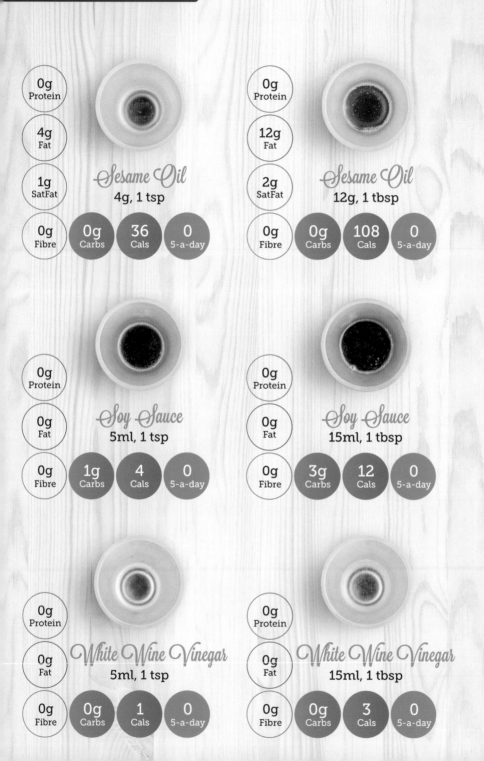

0g Protein
4g Fat
1g SatFat
0g Fibre

Sesame Oil
4g, 1 tsp

0g Carbs · 36 Cals · 0 5-a-day

0g Protein
12g Fat
2g SatFat
0g Fibre

Sesame Oil
12g, 1 tbsp

0g Carbs · 108 Cals · 0 5-a-day

0g Protein
0g Fat
0g Fibre

Soy Sauce
5ml, 1 tsp

1g Carbs · 4 Cals · 0 5-a-day

0g Protein
0g Fat
0g Fibre

Soy Sauce
15ml, 1 tbsp

3g Carbs · 12 Cals · 0 5-a-day

0g Protein
0g Fat
0g Fibre

White Wine Vinegar
5ml, 1 tsp

0g Carbs · 1 Cals · 0 5-a-day

0g Protein
0g Fat
0g Fibre

White Wine Vinegar
15ml, 1 tbsp

0g Carbs · 3 Cals · 0 5-a-day

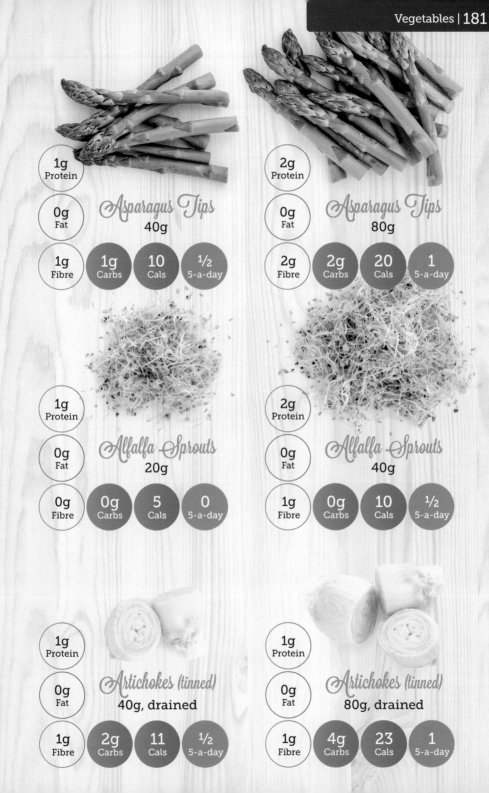

1g Protein

0g Fat

1g Fibre

Asparagus Tips
40g

1g Carbs · **10** Cals · **½** 5-a-day

2g Protein

0g Fat

2g Fibre

Asparagus Tips
80g

2g Carbs · **20** Cals · **1** 5-a-day

1g Protein

0g Fat

0g Fibre

Alfalfa Sprouts
20g

0g Carbs · **5** Cals · **0** 5-a-day

2g Protein

0g Fat

1g Fibre

Alfalfa Sprouts
40g

0g Carbs · **10** Cals · **½** 5-a-day

1g Protein

0g Fat

1g Fibre

Artichokes (tinned)
40g, drained

2g Carbs · **11** Cals · **½** 5-a-day

1g Protein

0g Fat

1g Fibre

Artichokes (tinned)
80g, drained

4g Carbs · **23** Cals · **1** 5-a-day

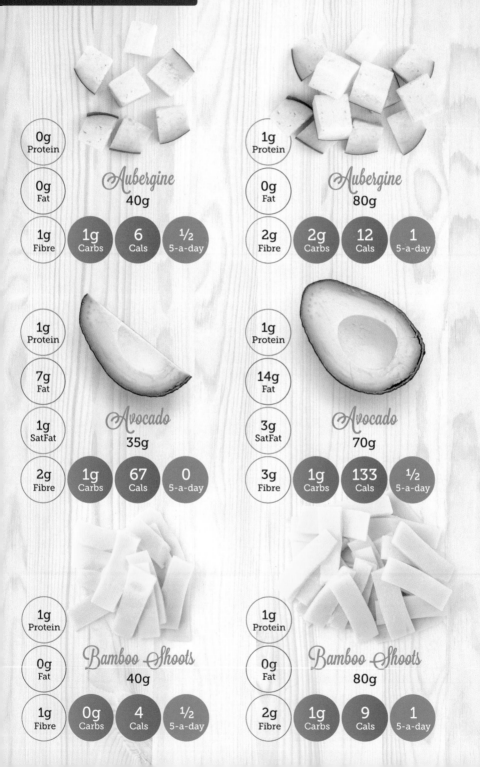

Aubergine
40g

0g Protein

0g Fat

1g Fibre

1g Carbs

6 Cals

½ 5-a-day

Aubergine
80g

1g Protein

0g Fat

2g Fibre

2g Carbs

12 Cals

1 5-a-day

Avocado
35g

1g Protein

7g Fat

1g SatFat

2g Fibre

1g Carbs

67 Cals

0 5-a-day

Avocado
70g

1g Protein

14g Fat

3g SatFat

3g Fibre

1g Carbs

133 Cals

½ 5-a-day

Bamboo Shoots
40g

1g Protein

0g Fat

1g Fibre

0g Carbs

4 Cals

½ 5-a-day

Bamboo Shoots
80g

1g Protein

0g Fat

2g Fibre

1g Carbs

9 Cals

1 5-a-day

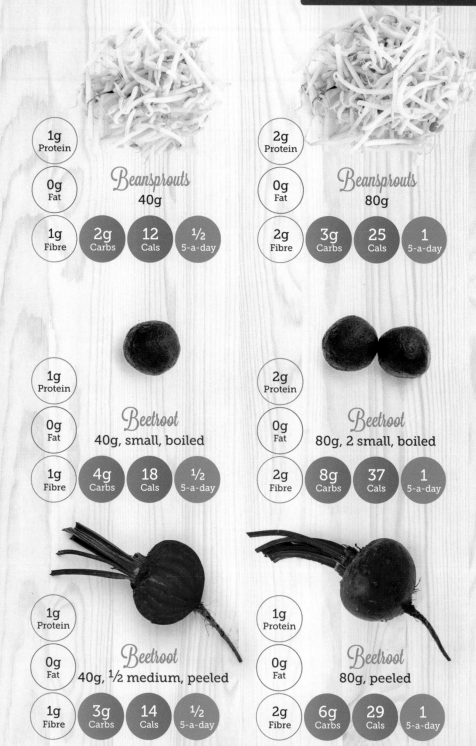

Beansprouts
40g

1g Protein
0g Fat
1g Fibre
2g Carbs
12 Cals
½ 5-a-day

Beansprouts
80g

2g Protein
0g Fat
2g Fibre
3g Carbs
25 Cals
1 5-a-day

Beetroot
40g, small, boiled

1g Protein
0g Fat
1g Fibre
4g Carbs
18 Cals
½ 5-a-day

Beetroot
80g, 2 small, boiled

2g Protein
0g Fat
2g Fibre
8g Carbs
37 Cals
1 5-a-day

Beetroot
40g, ½ medium, peeled

1g Protein
0g Fat
1g Fibre
3g Carbs
14 Cals
½ 5-a-day

Beetroot
80g, peeled

1g Protein
0g Fat
2g Fibre
6g Carbs
29 Cals
1 5-a-day

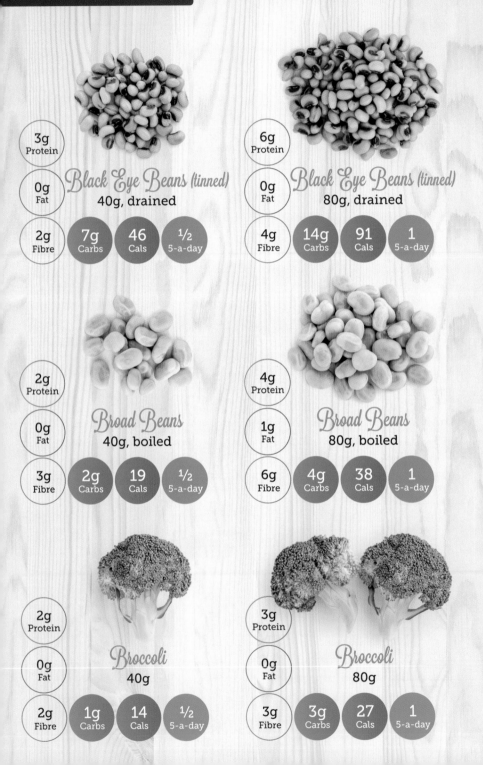

Black Eye Beans (tinned)
40g, drained

3g Protein
0g Fat
2g Fibre
7g Carbs
46 Cals
½ 5-a-day

Black Eye Beans (tinned)
80g, drained

6g Protein
0g Fat
4g Fibre
14g Carbs
91 Cals
1 5-a-day

Broad Beans
40g, boiled

2g Protein
0g Fat
3g Fibre
2g Carbs
19 Cals
½ 5-a-day

Broad Beans
80g, boiled

4g Protein
1g Fat
6g Fibre
4g Carbs
38 Cals
1 5-a-day

Broccoli
40g

2g Protein
0g Fat
2g Fibre
1g Carbs
14 Cals
½ 5-a-day

Broccoli
80g

3g Protein
0g Fat
3g Fibre
3g Carbs
27 Cals
1 5-a-day

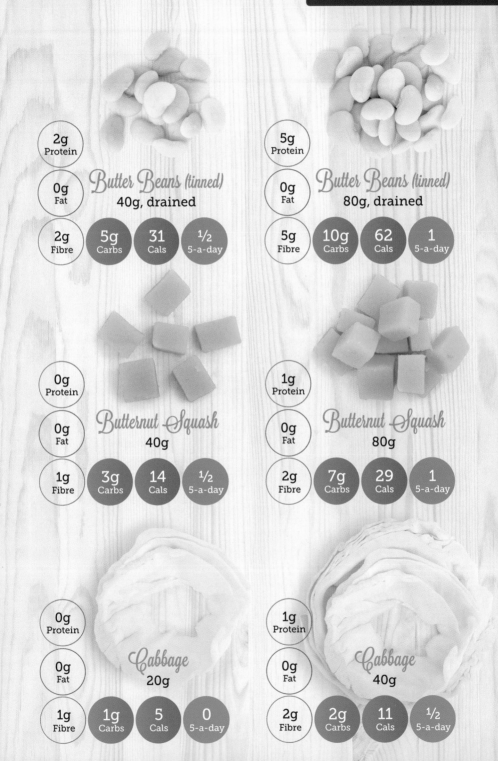

2g Protein

0g Fat

2g Fibre

Butter Beans (tinned)
40g, drained

5g Carbs · 31 Cals · ½ 5-a-day

5g Protein

0g Fat

5g Fibre

Butter Beans (tinned)
80g, drained

10g Carbs · 62 Cals · 1 5-a-day

0g Protein

0g Fat

1g Fibre

Butternut Squash
40g

3g Carbs · 14 Cals · ½ 5-a-day

1g Protein

0g Fat

2g Fibre

Butternut Squash
80g

7g Carbs · 29 Cals · 1 5-a-day

0g Protein

0g Fat

1g Fibre

Cabbage
20g

1g Carbs · 5 Cals · 0 5-a-day

1g Protein

0g Fat

2g Fibre

Cabbage
40g

2g Carbs · 11 Cals · ½ 5-a-day

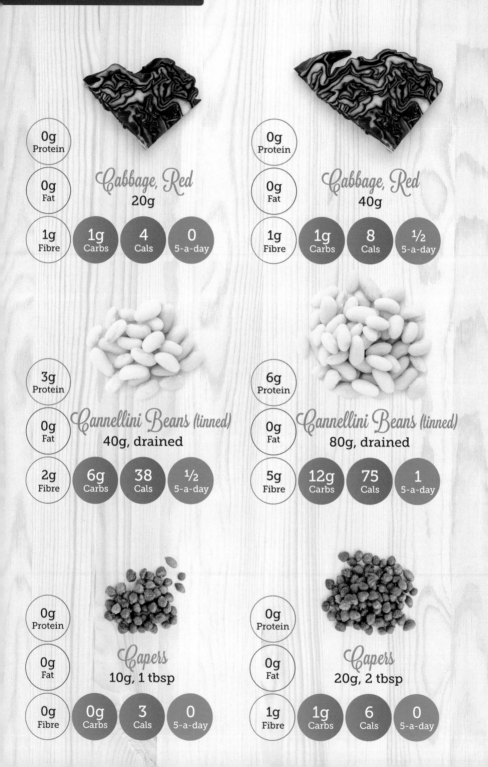

Protein	0g
Fat	0g
Fibre	1g

Cabbage, Red
20g

| 1g Carbs | 4 Cals | 0 5-a-day |

Protein	0g
Fat	0g
Fibre	1g

Cabbage, Red
40g

| 1g Carbs | 8 Cals | ½ 5-a-day |

Protein	3g
Fat	0g
Fibre	2g

Cannellini Beans (tinned)
40g, drained

| 6g Carbs | 38 Cals | ½ 5-a-day |

Protein	6g
Fat	0g
Fibre	5g

Cannellini Beans (tinned)
80g, drained

| 12g Carbs | 75 Cals | 1 5-a-day |

Protein	0g
Fat	0g
Fibre	0g

Capers
10g, 1 tbsp

| 0g Carbs | 3 Cals | 0 5-a-day |

Protein	0g
Fat	0g
Fibre	1g

Capers
20g, 2 tbsp

| 1g Carbs | 6 Cals | 0 5-a-day |

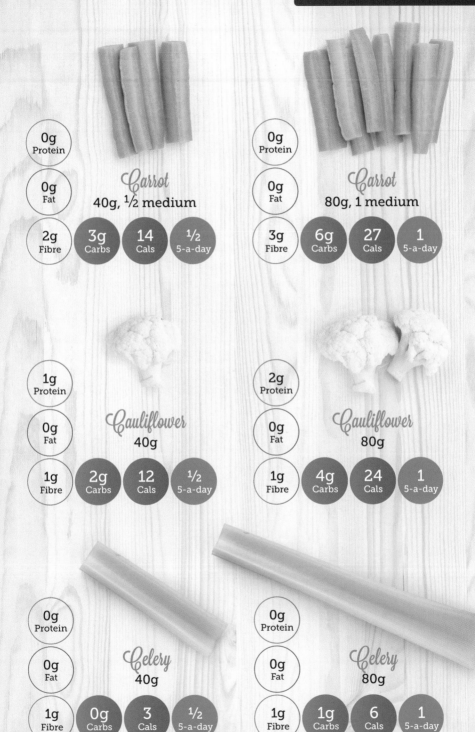

0g
Protein

0g
Fat

Carrot
40g, ½ medium

2g
Fibre

3g
Carbs

14
Cals

½
5-a-day

0g
Protein

0g
Fat

Carrot
80g, 1 medium

3g
Fibre

6g
Carbs

27
Cals

1
5-a-day

1g
Protein

0g
Fat

Cauliflower
40g

1g
Fibre

2g
Carbs

12
Cals

½
5-a-day

2g
Protein

0g
Fat

Cauliflower
80g

1g
Fibre

4g
Carbs

24
Cals

1
5-a-day

0g
Protein

0g
Fat

Celery
40g

1g
Fibre

0g
Carbs

3
Cals

½
5-a-day

0g
Protein

0g
Fat

Celery
80g

1g
Fibre

1g
Carbs

6
Cals

1
5-a-day

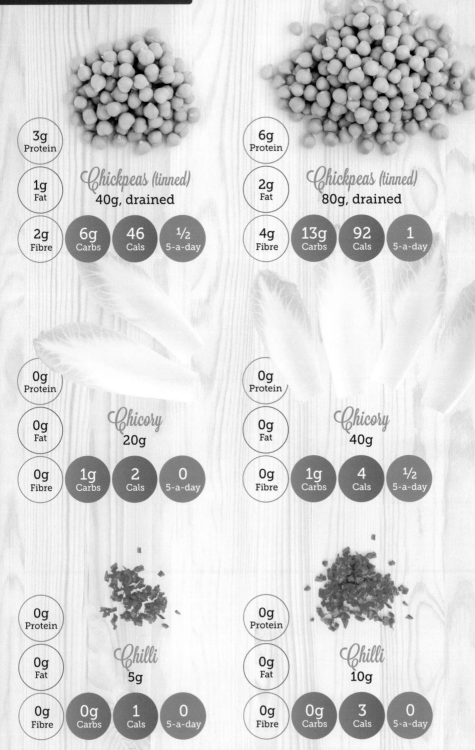

3g Protein
1g Fat
2g Fibre

Chickpeas (tinned)
40g, drained

6g Carbs
46 Cals
½ 5-a-day

6g Protein
2g Fat
4g Fibre

Chickpeas (tinned)
80g, drained

13g Carbs
92 Cals
1 5-a-day

0g Protein
0g Fat
0g Fibre

Chicory
20g

1g Carbs
2 Cals
0 5-a-day

0g Protein
0g Fat
0g Fibre

Chicory
40g

1g Carbs
4 Cals
½ 5-a-day

0g Protein
0g Fat
0g Fibre

Chilli
5g

0g Carbs
1 Cals
0 5-a-day

0g Protein
0g Fat
0g Fibre

Chilli
10g

0g Carbs
3 Cals
0 5-a-day

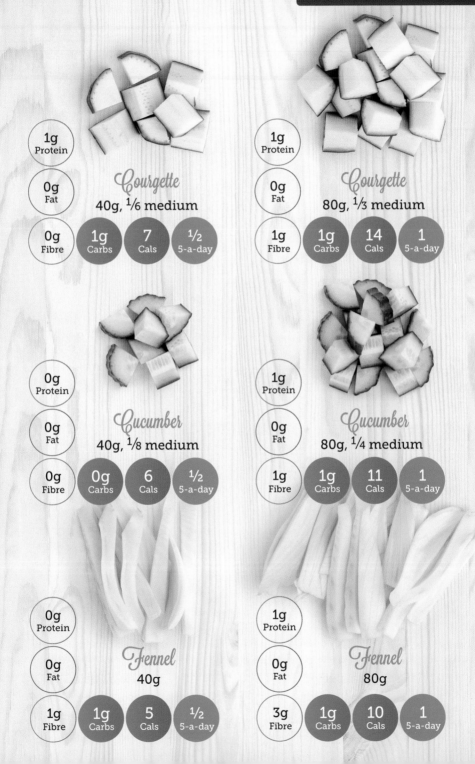

1g
Protein

0g
Fat

0g
Fibre

Courgette
40g, ¹/₆ medium

1g
Carbs

7
Cals

¹/₂
5-a-day

1g
Protein

0g
Fat

1g
Fibre

Courgette
80g, ¹/₃ medium

1g
Carbs

14
Cals

1
5-a-day

0g
Protein

0g
Fat

0g
Fibre

Cucumber
40g, ¹/₈ medium

0g
Carbs

6
Cals

¹/₂
5-a-day

1g
Protein

0g
Fat

1g
Fibre

Cucumber
80g, ¹/₄ medium

1g
Carbs

11
Cals

1
5-a-day

0g
Protein

0g
Fat

1g
Fibre

Fennel
40g

1g
Carbs

5
Cals

¹/₂
5-a-day

1g
Protein

0g
Fat

3g
Fibre

Fennel
80g

1g
Carbs

10
Cals

1
5-a-day

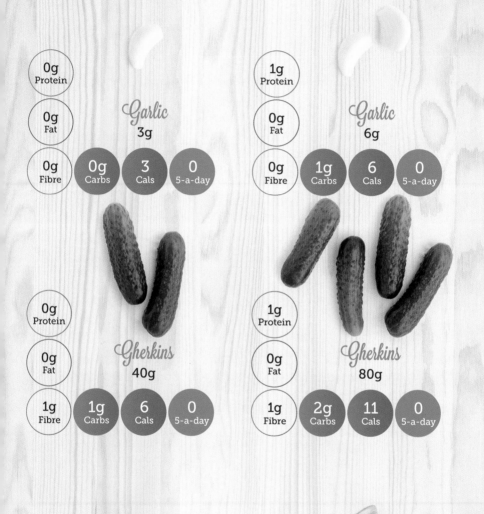

0g Protein			
0g Fat	**Garlic** 3g		
0g Fibre	0g Carbs	3 Cals	0 5-a-day

1g Protein			
0g Fat	**Garlic** 6g		
0g Fibre	1g Carbs	6 Cals	0 5-a-day

0g Protein			
0g Fat	**Gherkins** 40g		
1g Fibre	1g Carbs	6 Cals	0 5-a-day

1g Protein			
0g Fat	**Gherkins** 80g		
1g Fibre	2g Carbs	11 Cals	0 5-a-day

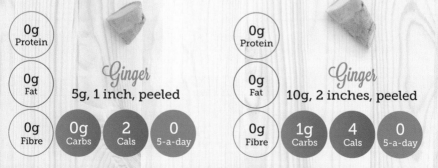

0g Protein			
0g Fat	**Ginger** 5g, 1 inch, peeled		
0g Fibre	0g Carbs	2 Cals	0 5-a-day

0g Protein			
0g Fat	**Ginger** 10g, 2 inches, peeled		
0g Fibre	1g Carbs	4 Cals	0 5-a-day

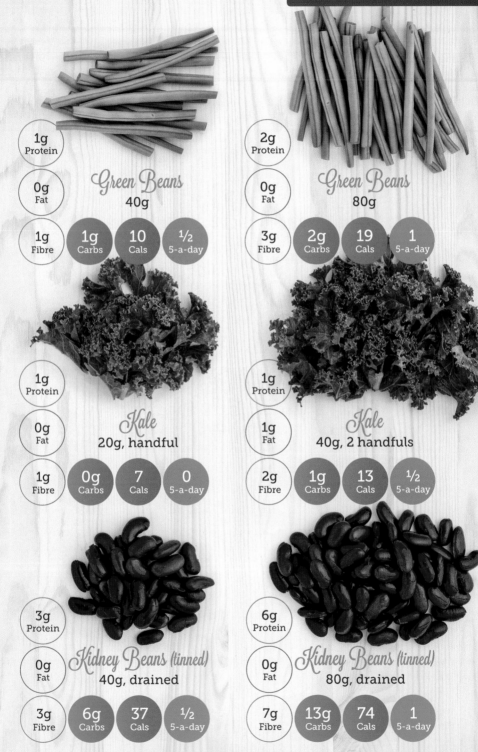

1g Protein

0g Fat

1g Fibre

Green Beans
40g

1g Carbs | **10** Cals | **½** 5-a-day

2g Protein

0g Fat

3g Fibre

Green Beans
80g

2g Carbs | **19** Cals | **1** 5-a-day

1g Protein

0g Fat

1g Fibre

Kale
20g, handful

0g Carbs | **7** Cals | **0** 5-a-day

1g Protein

1g Fat

2g Fibre

Kale
40g, 2 handfuls

1g Carbs | **13** Cals | **½** 5-a-day

3g Protein

0g Fat

3g Fibre

Kidney Beans (tinned)
40g, drained

6g Carbs | **37** Cals | **½** 5-a-day

6g Protein

0g Fat

7g Fibre

Kidney Beans (tinned)
80g, drained

13g Carbs | **74** Cals | **1** 5-a-day

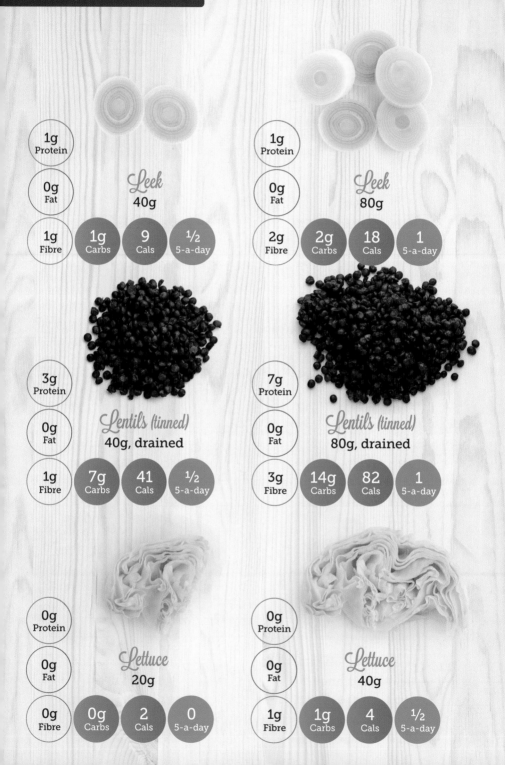

1g Protein			
0g Fat	*Leek* 40g		
1g Fibre	**1g** Carbs	**9** Cals	**½** 5-a-day

1g Protein			
0g Fat	*Leek* 80g		
2g Fibre	**2g** Carbs	**18** Cals	**1** 5-a-day

3g Protein			
0g Fat	*Lentils (tinned)* 40g, drained		
1g Fibre	**7g** Carbs	**41** Cals	**½** 5-a-day

7g Protein			
0g Fat	*Lentils (tinned)* 80g, drained		
3g Fibre	**14g** Carbs	**82** Cals	**1** 5-a-day

0g Protein			
0g Fat	*Lettuce* 20g		
0g Fibre	**0g** Carbs	**2** Cals	**0** 5-a-day

0g Protein			
0g Fat	*Lettuce* 40g		
1g Fibre	**1g** Carbs	**4** Cals	**½** 5-a-day

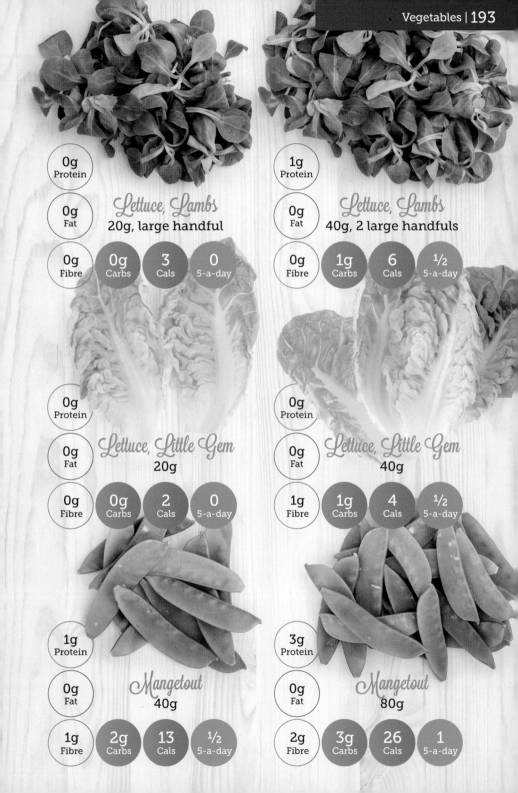

Lettuce, Lambs
20g, large handful

Protein	Fat	Fibre	Carbs	Cals	5-a-day
0g	0g	0g	0g	3	0

Lettuce, Lambs
40g, 2 large handfuls

Protein	Fat	Fibre	Carbs	Cals	5-a-day
1g	0g	0g	1g	6	½

Lettuce, Little Gem
20g

Protein	Fat	Fibre	Carbs	Cals	5-a-day
0g	0g	0g	0g	2	0

Lettuce, Little Gem
40g

Protein	Fat	Fibre	Carbs	Cals	5-a-day
0g	0g	1g	1g	4	½

Mangetout
40g

Protein	Fat	Fibre	Carbs	Cals	5-a-day
1g	0g	1g	2g	13	½

Mangetout
80g

Protein	Fat	Fibre	Carbs	Cals	5-a-day
3g	0g	2g	3g	26	1

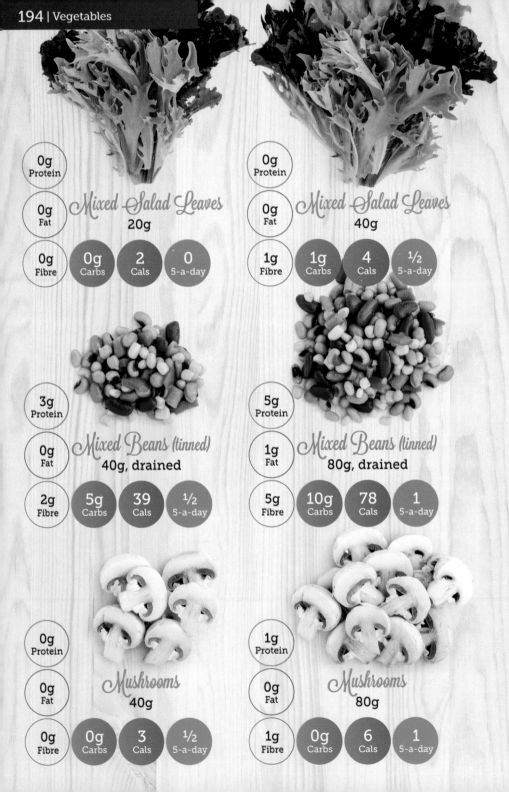

Mixed Salad Leaves
20g

0g Protein		
0g Fat		
0g Fibre	0g Carbs	2 Cals	0 5-a-day

Mixed Salad Leaves
40g

0g Protein		
0g Fat		
1g Fibre	1g Carbs	4 Cals	½ 5-a-day

Mixed Beans (tinned)
40g, drained

3g Protein		
0g Fat		
2g Fibre	5g Carbs	39 Cals	½ 5-a-day

Mixed Beans (tinned)
80g, drained

5g Protein		
1g Fat		
5g Fibre	10g Carbs	78 Cals	1 5-a-day

Mushrooms
40g

0g Protein		
0g Fat		
0g Fibre	0g Carbs	3 Cals	½ 5-a-day

Mushrooms
80g

1g Protein		
0g Fat		
1g Fibre	0g Carbs	6 Cals	1 5-a-day

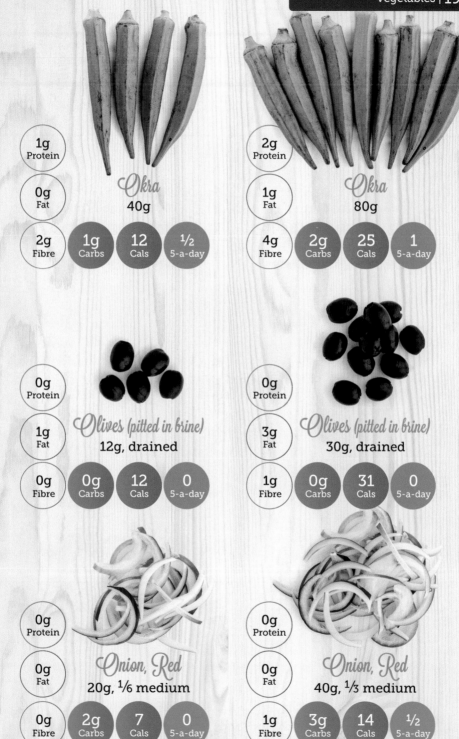

1g Protein
0g Fat
2g Fibre

Okra
40g

1g Carbs
12 Cals
½ 5-a-day

2g Protein
1g Fat
4g Fibre

Okra
80g

2g Carbs
25 Cals
1 5-a-day

0g Protein
1g Fat
0g Fibre

Olives (pitted in brine)
12g, drained

0g Carbs
12 Cals
0 5-a-day

0g Protein
3g Fat
1g Fibre

Olives (pitted in brine)
30g, drained

0g Carbs
31 Cals
0 5-a-day

0g Protein
0g Fat
0g Fibre

Onion, Red
20g, ⅙ medium

2g Carbs
7 Cals
0 5-a-day

0g Protein
0g Fat
1g Fibre

Onion, Red
40g, ⅓ medium

3g Carbs
14 Cals
½ 5-a-day

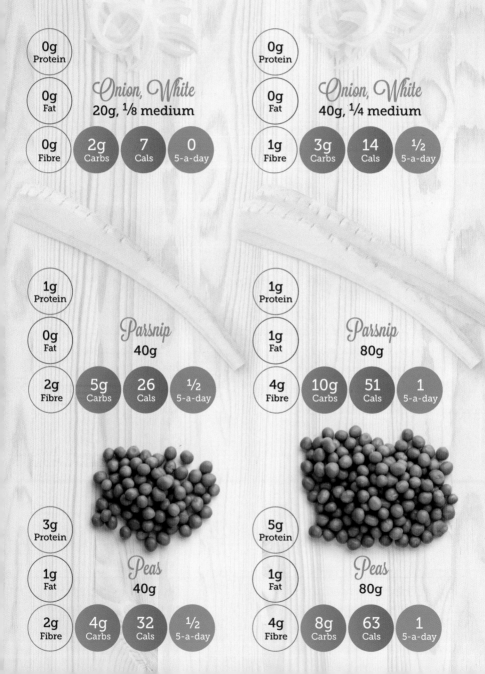

0g Protein
0g Fat
0g Fibre

Onion, White
20g, 1/8 medium

2g Carbs
7 Cals
0 5-a-day

0g Protein
0g Fat
1g Fibre

Onion, White
40g, 1/4 medium

3g Carbs
14 Cals
1/2 5-a-day

1g Protein
0g Fat
2g Fibre

Parsnip
40g

5g Carbs
26 Cals
1/2 5-a-day

1g Protein
1g Fat
4g Fibre

Parsnip
80g

10g Carbs
51 Cals
1 5-a-day

3g Protein
1g Fat
2g Fibre

Peas
40g

4g Carbs
32 Cals
1/2 5-a-day

5g Protein
1g Fat
4g Fibre

Peas
80g

8g Carbs
63 Cals
1 5-a-day

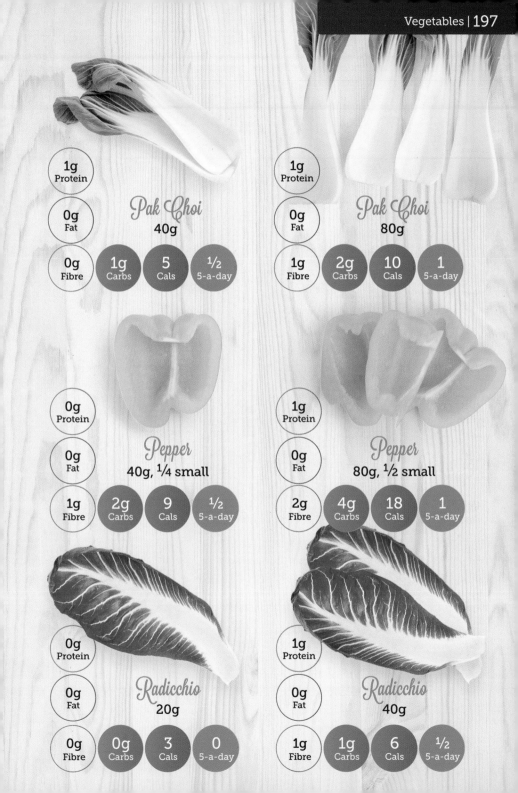

Pak Choi
40g

- 1g Protein
- 0g Fat
- 0g Fibre
- 1g Carbs
- 5 Cals
- ½ 5-a-day

Pak Choi
80g

- 1g Protein
- 0g Fat
- 1g Fibre
- 2g Carbs
- 10 Cals
- 1 5-a-day

Pepper
40g, ¼ small

- 0g Protein
- 0g Fat
- 1g Fibre
- 2g Carbs
- 9 Cals
- ½ 5-a-day

Pepper
80g, ½ small

- 1g Protein
- 0g Fat
- 2g Fibre
- 4g Carbs
- 18 Cals
- 1 5-a-day

Radicchio
20g

- 0g Protein
- 0g Fat
- 0g Fibre
- 0g Carbs
- 3 Cals
- 0 5-a-day

Radicchio
40g

- 1g Protein
- 0g Fat
- 1g Fibre
- 1g Carbs
- 6 Cals
- ½ 5-a-day

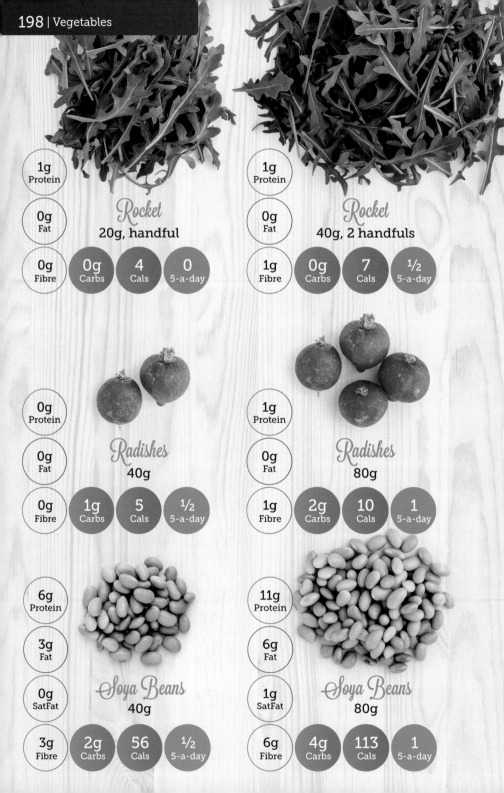

Rocket
20g, handful

1g Protein	0g Fat	0g Fibre

0g Carbs	4 Cals	0 5-a-day

Rocket
40g, 2 handfuls

1g Protein	0g Fat	1g Fibre

0g Carbs	7 Cals	½ 5-a-day

Radishes
40g

0g Protein	0g Fat	0g Fibre

1g Carbs	5 Cals	½ 5-a-day

Radishes
80g

1g Protein	0g Fat	1g Fibre

2g Carbs	10 Cals	1 5-a-day

Soya Beans
40g

6g Protein	3g Fat	0g SatFat	3g Fibre

2g Carbs	56 Cals	½ 5-a-day

Soya Beans
80g

11g Protein	6g Fat	1g SatFat	6g Fibre

4g Carbs	113 Cals	1 5-a-day

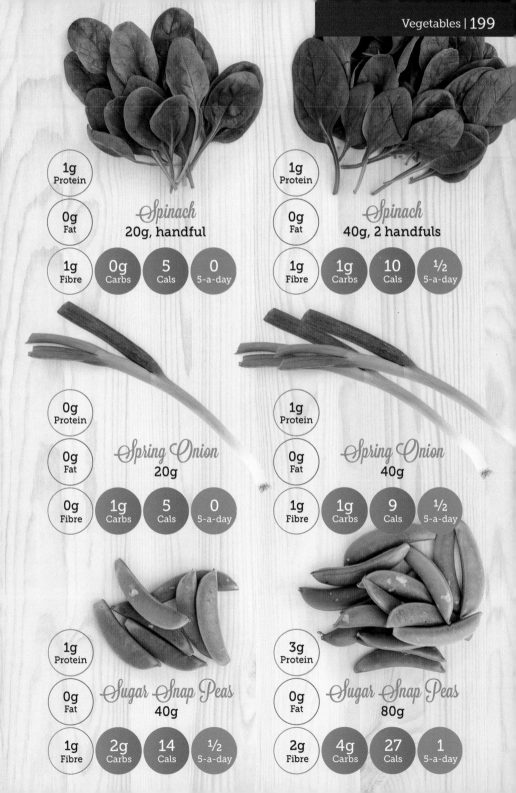

Spinach
20g, handful

1g Protein
0g Fat
1g Fibre
0g Carbs
5 Cals
0 5-a-day

Spinach
40g, 2 handfuls

1g Protein
0g Fat
1g Fibre
1g Carbs
10 Cals
½ 5-a-day

Spring Onion
20g

0g Protein
0g Fat
0g Fibre
1g Carbs
5 Cals
0 5-a-day

Spring Onion
40g

1g Protein
0g Fat
1g Fibre
1g Carbs
9 Cals
½ 5-a-day

Sugar Snap Peas
40g

1g Protein
0g Fat
1g Fibre
2g Carbs
14 Cals
½ 5-a-day

Sugar Snap Peas
80g

3g Protein
0g Fat
2g Fibre
4g Carbs
27 Cals
1 5-a-day

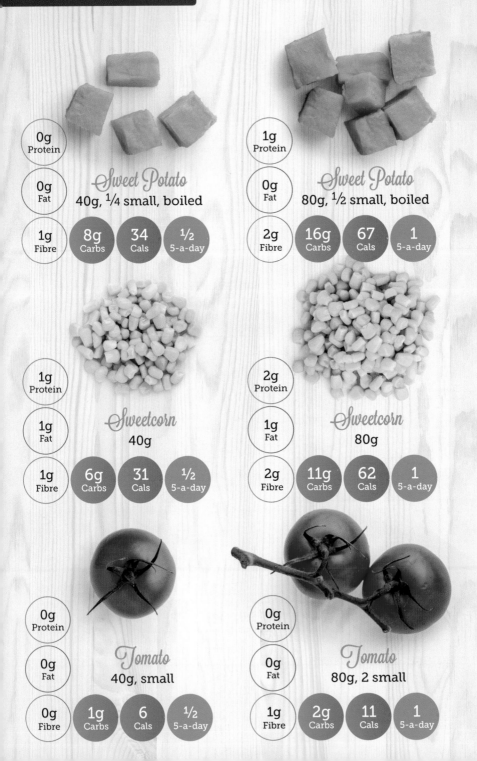

Sweet Potato
40g, ¼ small, boiled

0g Protein
0g Fat
1g Fibre
8g Carbs
34 Cals
½ 5-a-day

Sweet Potato
80g, ½ small, boiled

1g Protein
0g Fat
2g Fibre
16g Carbs
67 Cals
1 5-a-day

Sweetcorn
40g

1g Protein
1g Fat
1g Fibre
6g Carbs
31 Cals
½ 5-a-day

Sweetcorn
80g

2g Protein
1g Fat
2g Fibre
11g Carbs
62 Cals
1 5-a-day

Tomato
40g, small

0g Protein
0g Fat
0g Fibre
1g Carbs
6 Cals
½ 5-a-day

Tomato
80g, 2 small

0g Protein
0g Fat
1g Fibre
2g Carbs
11 Cals
1 5-a-day

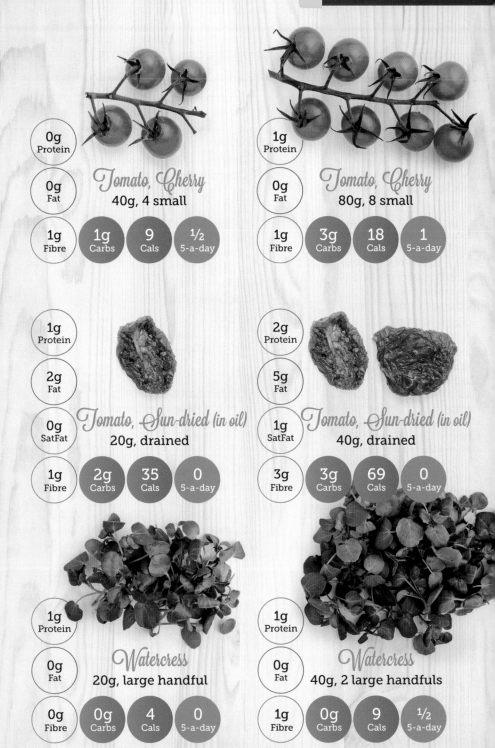

0g Protein

0g Fat

1g Fibre

Tomato, Cherry
40g, 4 small

1g Carbs | **9** Cals | **½** 5-a-day

1g Protein

0g Fat

1g Fibre

Tomato, Cherry
80g, 8 small

3g Carbs | **18** Cals | **1** 5-a-day

1g Protein

2g Fat

0g SatFat

1g Fibre

Tomato, Sun-dried (in oil)
20g, drained

2g Carbs | **35** Cals | **0** 5-a-day

2g Protein

5g Fat

1g SatFat

3g Fibre

Tomato, Sun-dried (in oil)
40g, drained

3g Carbs | **69** Cals | **0** 5-a-day

1g Protein

0g Fat

0g Fibre

Watercress
20g, large handful

0g Carbs | **4** Cals | **0** 5-a-day

1g Protein

0g Fat

1g Fibre

Watercress
40g, 2 large handfuls

0g Carbs | **9** Cals | **½** 5-a-day

Recipes

Ingredients

About the Authors

Chris Cheyette BSc (Hons) MSc RD
Diabetes Specialist Dietitian

Chris is a Diabetes Specialist Dietitian within the NHS, working with people with type 1, type 2 and gestational diabetes. Chris has spearheaded a number of projects over the years, many with the aim of improving diabetes educational resources. These include an educational DVD for young people with diabetes, which earned him the 2007 British Dietetic Association Elizabeth Washington Award. Chris has also published a number of journal articles on weight management and diabetes. He regularly undertakes local and national presentations to healthcare professionals, has done TV & newspaper interviews, and has participated as a guest expert in online discussions.

Yello Balolia BA (Hons)
Entrepreneur & Creative Photographer

Having achieved a first class honours degree in Photography, Canada-born, Blackpool-bred and now London-based Yello used his entrepreneurial and creative skills to found Chello Publishing Limited with Chris Cheyette, to publish Carbs & Cals (**www.carbsandcals.com**), the bestselling and multi-award-winning book and app for diabetes and weight management. He has also undertaken a series of creative projects including private commissions (**www.yellobalolia.com**) and, as a keen musician, Yello recently set up Ukulology - a visual and effective way of learning the ukulele (**www.ukulology.com**).

Awards

Carbs & Cals won **Best Dietary Management Initiative** at the Quality in Care Awards 2014

The Carbs & Cals App won **New Product of the Year** in the Complete Nutrition Awards 2012

Carbs & Cals won the BDA Dame Barbara Clayton **Award for Innovation & Excellence** 2011

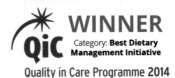

WINNER
Category: **Best Dietary Management Initiative**
Quality in Care Programme 2014

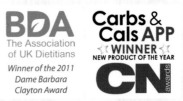

BDA
The Association of UK Dietitians
Winner of the 2011 Dame Barbara Clayton Award

Carbs & Cals APP
WINNER
NEW PRODUCT OF THE YEAR

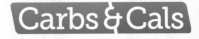

Carbs & Cals